Current and Future Application of Artificial Intelligence in Clinical Medicine

Edited by

Shigao Huang

Faculty of Health Science,
University of Macau,
Macau,
China

&

Jie Yang

Department of Computer and Information Science,
University of Macau,
Macau,
China

Current and Future Application of Artificial Intelligence in Clinical Medicine

Editors: Shigao Huang and Jie Yang

ISBN (Online): 978-1-68108-841-9

ISBN (Print): 978-1-68108-842-6

ISBN (Paperback): 978-1-68108-843-3

Published by Bentham Science Publishers – Sharjah, UAE. All Rights Reserved.

need for a court order if at any point you breach any terms of this License Agreement. In no event will any delay or failure by Bentham Science Publishers in enforcing your compliance with this License Agreement constitute a waiver of any of its rights.

3. You acknowledge that you have read this License Agreement, and agree to be bound by its terms and conditions. To the extent that any other terms and conditions presented on any website of Bentham Science Publishers conflict with, or are inconsistent with, the terms and conditions set out in this License Agreement, you acknowledge that the terms and conditions set out in this License Agreement shall prevail.

Bentham Science Publishers Ltd.
Executive Suite Y - 2
PO Box 7917, Saif Zone
Sharjah, U.A.E.
Email: subscriptions@benthamscience.net

BENTHAM SCIENCE

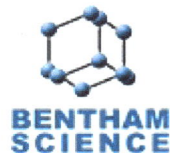

CONTENTS

PREFACE

Artificial intelligence (AI) brought me a breakthrough regarding clinical data and computer models. Nowadays, with the development of AI significantly advances progress, we hope the researcher can utilize this modern technology to improve clinical accuracy such as diagnosis, prognosis, therapeutic, and so on. Clinical work is filled enough with patients and they need AI help to minimize workload and improve the high efficiency of the medical assignment.

Titled "Current and Prevalent Trends in Clinical Medicine with Artificial Intelligence" this book included AI application in cancer diagnosis and prognosis, AI accelerates the development and transformation of the medical care AI in China's COVID-19 Pandemic and AI experience of fighting with the COVID-19. All readers welcome to read. In this book, you can learn the AI technology with Clinical knowledge., the latest advance of AI application in the clinic, even now, it can be applied in the COVID-19 pandemic. We are trying to collect the latest issue regarding AI in Clinical Oncology.

In preparing this book we have had the privilege of collaborating with outstanding contributors from leading comprehensive cancer and computer specialist. We believe that the authors' expertise, distinguished pieces of knowledge, and multidisciplinary approaches provide a valuable source of information and can guide decision-making for physicians and clinical researchers.

All physicians active in the field of cancer diagnosis and treatment (oncologists, oncologic surgeons, radiation oncologists, nuclear medicine physicians, and radiologists) and computer specialists on artificial intelligence are the target audience for this book. The book can also be used to train young specialists who are preparing for a multidisciplinary crossover examination.

We dedicate this book to those who treat people with dignity and respect and to organizations and individuals committed to building a peaceful world.

Shigao Huang
Faculty of Health Science
University of Macau
Macau
China

ACKNOWLEDGEMENT

Shaanxi Jiuzhou Biomedical Science and Technology Group referred to as "Jiuzhou Group", founded in September 2006, is located in Xi'an Hi-tech Development Zone in China established by Shaanxi Jiuzhou Biotechnology Co., Ltd. and Shaanxi high tech Industry Investment Co., Ltd. Main business: research and development and transformation of cell biotechnology, professional platform service of life science, precision medical diagnosis, medical service, health management, *etc*. Jiuzhou Group began to invest in the construction of Shaanxi Jiuzhou biomedical science and Technology Park (currently, knew as Shaanxi Jiuzhou stem cell science and Technology Industrial Park) in 2002, which is a provincial key construction project in the 11th five year plan. At the beginning of the 12th Five Year Plan period, the first industrial transformation platform of cell gene was built in China (2010), and the whole industrial chain of cell collection, storage, detection, production and preparation, clinical research and application was built. After ten years of accumulation, the industrial pattern of "one park, one chain and one center" has been formed in Jiuzhou stem cell science and Technology Industrial Park, whole industrial chain of cell biology and Jiuzhou medical center.

Xi 'an Zer Huier Education Technology Co., Ltd., founded in 2018, in China, is a professional institution focusing on medical and health examination and training and improving the professional ability of the pharmaceutical industry. The company has the most professional team of teachers, all the lecturers are from domestic and foreign professional colleges and universities. They not only have made a lot of achievements in the relevant fields, but also have a wealth of teaching experience, focusing on the systematic training of professionals in the field of health care, to provide more breadth, validity, and professional training services for the field of health care in China.

List of Contributors

Amara Dar	Institute of Chemistry, University of The Punjab, Lahore, Pakistan
Feng Wu	Zhuhai Institutes of Advanced Technology of the Chinese Academy of Sciences, Zhuhai, China
Han Wang	Faculty of Data Science, City University of Macau, Taipa, Macau, China Zhuhai Institutes of Advanced Technology of the Chinese Academy of Sciences, Zhuhai, China
Jie Yang	Department of Computer and Information Science, University of Macau, Macau, China Chongqing Industry & Trade Polytechnic, Chongqing, China
Kairong Duan	Department of Electrical Engineering and Computer Sciences, University of California, Berkeley, CA, USA Department of Computer and Information Science, University of Macau, Macau, China
Kexing Liu	Department of Computer and Information Science, University of Macau, Macau, China
Komal Hayat	Department of Chemistry, Quaid-i-Azam University, Islamabad, Pakistan
Kun Lan	Department of Computer and Information Science, University of Macau, Macau, China
Lijian Tan	Chongqing Industry & Trade Polytechnic, University of Macau, Chongqing, China
Gang Liu	Tourism College, Hainan University, Haikou, China
Parsa Mahmood Dar	Institute of Chinese Medicine, University of Macau, Macau, China
Quanyi Hu	Department of Computer and Information Science, University of Macau, Macau, China
Qichao Wang	School of International Relations, Xi'an International Studies University, Xi'an, China
Qun Song	Department of Computer and Information Science, University of Macau, Macau, China
Qi Zhao	Institute of Translational Medicine, Faculty of Health Sciences, University of Macau, Macau, China
Rui Tang	Department of Management Science and Information System, Faculty of Management and Economics, Kunming University of Science and Technology, Kunming, China
Shigao Huang	Institute of Translational Medicine, Faculty of Health Sciences, University of Macau, Macau, China
Simon Fong	Zhuhai Institutes of Advanced Technology of the Chinese Academy of Sciences, Zhuhai, China Department of Computer and Information Science, University of Macau, Macau, China

Sunny Yaoyang Wu Department of Computer and Information Science, University of Macau, Macau, China

Ting Gao Baoji Vocational and Technical College, Baoji, Shaan Xi, China

Tao Qi Department of Radiation Oncology, 986 Hospital of People's Liberation Army Air Force, Xi'an, Shaan Xi, P.R. China

Xianxian Liu Department of Computer and Information Science, University of Macau, Macau, China

Xiaoxia Li Shaanxi ZeEr HuiEr Education Technology Co. LTD, Shaanxi, Xi'an, China

CHAPTER 1

Artificial Intelligence (AI) in Cancer Diagnosis and Prognosis

Parsa Mahmood Dar[1,*], Amara Dar[2] and Komal Hayat[3]

[1] *Institute of Chinese Medicine, University of Macau, Macau, China*

[2] *Institute of Chemistry, University of The Punjab, Lahore, Pakistan*

[3] *Department of Chemistry, Quaid-i-Azam University, Islamabad, Pakistan*

Abstract: Cancer is a disorder with aggressive, low-median survival. Unfortunately, the healing time is long and expensive owing to high recurrence and mortality rates. It is essential to increase patient survival. Over the years, mathematical and computer engineering advancements have inspired numerous scientists to use quantitative methods to evaluate disease prognosis, such as multivariate statistical analysis, and the precision of these studies is considerably higher than that of observational predictions. However, as artificial intelligence (AI) has found widespread applications in clinical cancer research in recent years, especially machine learning and deep learning, cancer prediction output has reached new heights. The literature on the use of AI for cancer diagnosis and prognosis is discussed in this part. We discuss how AI supports the diagnosis of cancer, especially in terms of its unparalleled precision. We also illustrate forms in which these approaches progress the field. Opportunities and problems are addressed in the clinical application of AI.

Keywords: Artificial intelligence, Big data, Deep learning, Machine learning, Medical care.

1. INTRODUCTION

By allowing significant changes in communication, transportation, and media, Artificial Intelligence (AI) and Machine Learning (ML) have an enormous effect on our daily lives. AI has also recently achieved incredible heights in the science of clinical cancer. It is used to help in cancer diagnosis and prognosis, considering its unparalleled degree of sensitivity, far higher than that of a general statistical expert [1].

** **Corresponding author Parsa Mahmood Dar:** Institute of Chinese Medicine, University of Macau, Macau, China. Tel: 853 88222952, Fax: 853 88222952, E-mail: parsadar4@gmail.com

Shigao Huang and Jie Yang (Eds.)

The most complex disease condition of all is cancer, which may be malignant. Numbers for 2018 showed around 9.6 million cancer deaths worldwide. Although the incidence of cancer mortality from the US has been estimated to decrease by 27%, this evidence does not reassure the present estimates since the number of cases of cancer reported each year has not decreased [2]. Almost 1.7 million new cases of cancer were reported in 2019, and 0.6 million deaths were recorded. It is necessary to study and practise such clinical techniques that help minimise the likelihood of mortality, considering the current scenario. The technology of AI for healthcare reform flourishes every day. Large data can be learned and understood from this scientific breakthrough [3].

In the early stages, cancer is impossible to diagnose, and there are chances of recurrence after treatment. In comparison, precise, high-security disease predictions are very difficult. A simple search of the literature shows that the number of research papers on cancer has increased exponentially, especially those involving AI tools and large databases containing historical clinical cases for AI models [4]. In retrospective trials, the common approach is to obtain basic clinical results along through the use of the traditional TNM staging system (based on tumour size (T), the spread of cancer to nearby lymph nodes (N), and the spread of cancer to other parts of the body (M, for metastasis), yet incorrect prognosis seems to be a bottleneck for clinicians [5].

Given the importance of time for cancer patients, AI has been widely used in clinical cancer studies over the years due to its usefulness and advantages. The present study selected and analysed PubMed, Google Scholar, CNKI, and WANFANG datasets from 1995-2019. Using matching keywords, 3594 papers were identified to be related to AI cancer studies in these databases. One thousand one hundred thirty-six documents, from a total of 2458 papers, were found similar and deleted. These papers were further examined for relevance using their headings/abstracts, and 2365 papers were deemed significant. We included 126 full-text papers on cancer detection and prognosis utilizing AI using a forward citation search [6].

As vast numbers of cancer-diagnosed patients and those who have endured multiple treatments have accrued through the years, it is possible that early cancer diagnosis will be improved using this archive.

2. MAJOR CANCER TYPE

Men are mostly vulnerable to prostate, colorectal, and lung cancers. Together, they account for 42 percent of all diagnoses in adults, with almost 1 in 5 new cases of prostate cancer alone.

For women, breast, prostate, and colorectal cancer are the three most prevalent cancers. Together, they account for half of all incidents, with 30% of new cases of breast cancer alone.

Such malignancies also blame for the largest number of casualties. Lung cancer accounts for almost one-quarter of all cancer deaths recorded worldwide. Data published by ourworldindata.org/cancer shows deaths reported by different cancers as well as internationally as shown in Fig. (**1**).

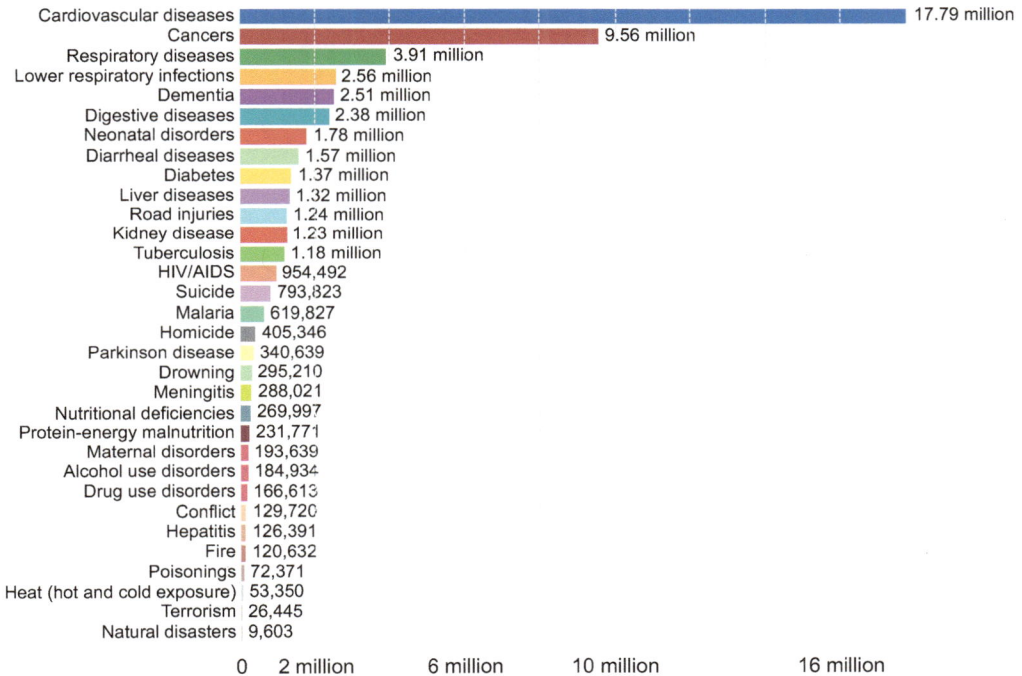

Fig. (1). Death caused globally due to cancers reported in 2017 [7].

2.1. Lung Cancer

Uncontrolled cell proliferation of lung tissues is the cause of lung cancer. From 1990 to 2016, mortality rates attributed to lung cancer decreased by 48 percent among men and 23 percent among women from 2002 to 2016. The number of new cases of lung cancer fell by 3 percent per year in men and 1.5 percent per year in women from 2011 to 2015. The disparities represent past trends in the usage of cigarettes, where several years later, women started smoking in significant numbers than women. Smoking habits do not seem to justify the higher lung cancer incidences recorded in women relative to men born around the 1960s [2] as shown in Fig. (**2**).

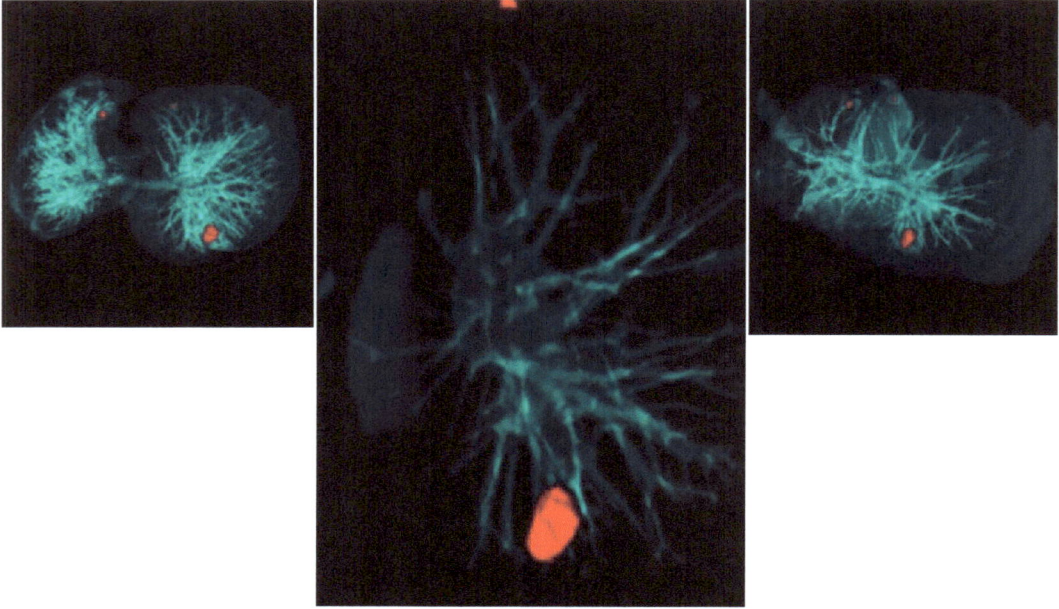

Fig. (2). Cancerous growth in lungs as diagnosed by AI [8]. An intelligent software system for lung cancer diagnostics has been developed by researchers from Peter the Great St.Petersburg Polytechnic University (SPbPU). The system analyzed anonymized CT images of 60 patients at the Oncological Center, and the focal nodules in lungs of small sizes (2 mm) could be successfully found.

2.2. Breast Cancer

Although breast cancer can occur in males and females, it is more potent in females. From 1989 to 2016, breast cancer mortality rates of women plunged 40%. This risk reduction is attributed to developments in early detection. The use of DNN as a breast cancer tool has been recorded with 96% precision [6] as shown in Fig. (3).

2.3. Prostate Cancer

It is the most prevalent type of cancer in men but not necessarily fatal. Many patients with prostate cancer die from this malignancy rather than collapse. Death rates for male prostate cancer dropped to 51% from 1993 till 2016. Owing to high over-diagnosis rates, routine screening with PSA blood testing is no longer recommended. Therefore, fewer prostate cancer reports are found [2] as shown in Fig. (4).

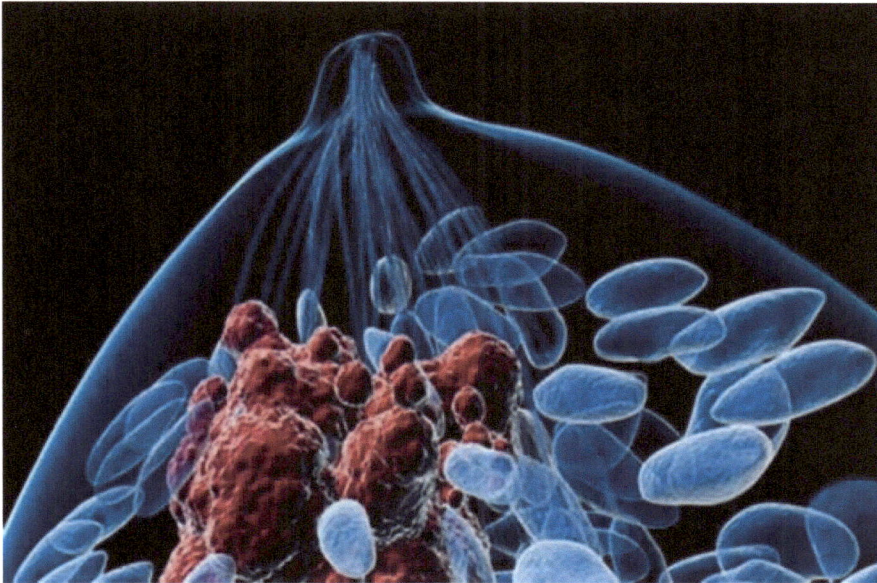

Fig. (3). Breast cancer imaging using AI [9]. IEEE fellow Karen Panetta has built an AI technology to distinguish breast cancer cells from non-cancer cells by analyzing biopsy images. If a cancer is present, the AI tool will also determine the grade of cancer.

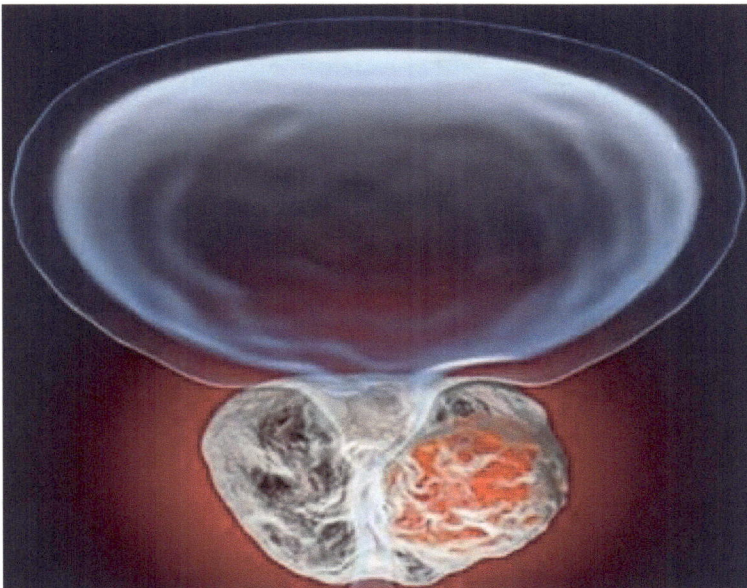

Fig. (4). AI helping early diagnosis of prostate cancer [10]. Radboud University Medical Center researchers have advanced a "deep learning" system that is more accurate than most pathologists in determining the aggressiveness of prostate cancer. The AI system, based on data from more than 1,200 patients, self-diagnoses itself to identify prostate cancer using tissue samples for diagnosis.

2.4. Colorectal Cancer

Colorectal cancer death rates declined by 53% from 1970 to 2016, thanks to increased screening and treatment advancements. Since the mid-1990s, however, new cases of colorectal cancer have increased by around 2 percent per year in people younger than age 55 [11] Fig. (**5**).

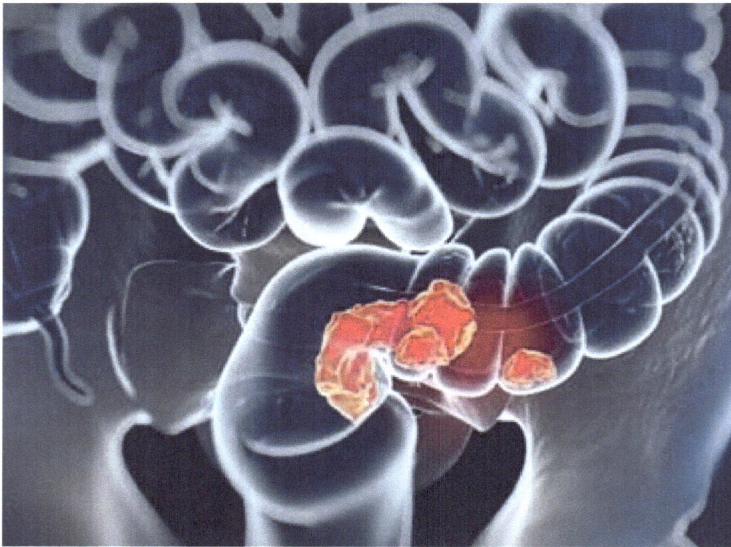

Fig. (5). Colorectal cancer diagnosis using AI [12]. AI has shown promising results in terms of accuracy in diagnosing CRC. However, the size and quality of training and validation datasets from most studies are relatively limited to apply the technology to clinical practice. In addition, external cross-validation is needed, especially for tumor classification.

2.5. Development in Diagnostic Tools

The decline in the death rate of cancer patients has been determined over time to be closely linked to early detection and adequate care [13]. The current technique is to use AI to achieve outcomes faster than the classical methods of diagnosis. The invention of the Virtual Reality Microscope (ARM) would continue to increase the functioning of the current procedure since it will be cost-effective, with readily accessible materials without the requirement for the study of whole slide graphical representations of the tissue.

Chinese researchers used detailed segmentation of brain tumours in AI and machine learning [14, 15]. For the detection of brain tumour and the assessment of surgical alternatives, tumour segmentation is important. Surgeons usually manually conduct personalised tumour segmentation, but their findings are not consistent. The results are correct, accurate, and reliable, preferring the usage of this established method.

SOPHiA GENETICS provides genomic software specifically developed to precisely classify the diverse mutational environment of large solid tumours such as lung, colorectal, skin, and brain cancers. They have licensed an AI-based cancer test kit that analyses patient DNA samples. It will accurately identify mutations/alterations in 42 genes related to solid cancers.

Tumours are either benign or malignant; not all tumours are cancerous. Recently, researchers from the University of Southern California's Viterbi School of Engineering have trained a machine-learning algorithm to distinguish between benign and malignant tumors for synthetic samples of breast cancer with an 80% accuracy rate.

In the study of the mammogram images and for the accurate diagnosis of breast cancer, Yala and his team evaluated and compared the diagnostic abilities of both the TC model and the coevolutionary neural network (new algorithm) and concluded that it dramatically enhanced risk discrimination [16].

Global developments in medical science in regions such as China, the USA, and Europe have demonstrated that AI requires time for adequate and prompt detection and detailed and reliable prognosis of deadly diseases such as cancer. Cancer prognosis provides estimates of recurrence of diseases and recovery of patients, with the goal of enhancing patient management [17, 18].

To evaluate the data collected from cancer patients, various mathematical models were used. By maintaining and reproducing the data, AI made the job simpler. Enshaei A *et al.* [19] contrasted a number of algorithms and classifiers with traditional statistical logistic regression approaches to demonstrate that AI may play a role in providing prognostic and predictive approaches.

3. ARTIFICIAL INTELLIGENCE (AI) IN PRECISION MEDICINE

Precision medicine theory operates on a customised patient care treatment approach based on the genomic understanding of the disease. This counselling method is not new, but patients with the same symptoms are usually treated on the same lines, ignoring the fact that each person has different responses due to different genetic compositions. A personalised medicinal approach that lets doctors select the patient's best treatment option is precision medicine or tailored medicine.

AI makes remarkable advances in drug discovery techniques, designing drugs, effectiveness of drugs' action, exposing molecular drug pathways, co-relating popular conditions, and analysing the most responsive patient population for a particular treatment. After 2016, various pharmaceutical corporations worldwide (such as Pfizer, IBM Watson, Exscientia) have partnered to develop active immune-modulating agents to give prospective patients new immune-oncology therapies. Exscientia, a UK-based company, leads the world of drug growth, researching various aspects of AI to create innovative medicines. They are the pioneers in drug synthesis process automation. GSK and Sanofi partnered with Exscientia to determine particular cancer goals and set specific medicines against these targets [20].

Table 1. AI applied to various kinds of cancer prognosis.

Type of Cancer	Methods of Study	Number of Patients in Study	Age of Patients (Years)	Year/ Region	Results	References
Breast Cancer	Multimodal DNN	1980	61	2018/ China	Not clear Conclusion	Sun *et al.* [21]
	Semi-supervised Learning Model	162500	N/A	2013/ USA	Not clear Conclusion	Park *et al.* [22]
	ANN and DT	433272	60.61	2005/ USA	Accuracy: DT (93.6%), ANN (91.2%)	Delen *et al.* [23]
	Dynamic Gradient Boosting	82707	58.38	2019/ USA	Accuracy Improved (28%)	Lu *et al.* [24]
Bladder Cancer	Statistical Analysis	115	N/A	2019/ China	NEDD8: Poor Prognosis Found	Tian *et al.* [25]
	KNN, RF, *etc*	3503	67.8	2019/ USA	Sensitivity& Specificity (> 70%)	Hasnain *et al.* [26]
Colorectal Cancer	Six Neural Networks	334	N/A	1997/ UK	Accuracy (> 80%), mean Sensitivity (60%),	Bottaci *et al.* [27]
	Semi-random Regression Tree	1568	N/A	2019/ China	/	Wang *et al.* [28]
	LSTM, Naïve Bayes, SVM	641	N/A	2018/ Finland	Hazard Ratio(2.3); CI(95%,1.79–3.03), AUC(0.69)	Bychkov *et al.* [29]

(Table 1) cont.....

Type of Cancer	Methods of Study	Number of Patients in Study	Age of Patients (Years)	Year/ Region	Results	References
Gastric Cancer	Cox Proportional Hazard, ANN	436	58.43 ± 13.02	2011/ Iran	TP(83.1%),	Biglarian *et al.* [30]
	ANN	289	63.20 ± 10.75	2013/ China	TP: ANN(85.3%)	Zhu *et al.* [31]
Glioma	Improved SVM	456	N/A	2018/ Taiwan	Accuracy(81.8%), ROC(0.922)	Lu *et al.* [32]
	GA and Nelder–Mead ML	70	48±15	2018/ Austria	Sensitivity (86%–98%), Specificity (92%–95%)	Papp *et al.* [33]
Long Bone Metastases	Multiple Additive Regression Trees	927	62±13	2015/ USA	-	Stein *et al.* [34]
Lung Cancer	GBM, SVM	10442	N/A	2017/ USA	RMSE (32,15.05) for GBM, SVM	Lynch *et al.* [35]
	SVM with RFE and RF	101	N/A	2018/ France	Accuracy (71%, 59%)	Sepehri *et al.* [36]
	Naive Bayes, SVM with Gaussian,	168	N/A	2016/ Italy	-	Yu *et al.* [37]
Oral Cavity Squamous Cell	RF, SVM	115	61.0 ± 12.	2017/ USA	AUC (0.72), Accuracy (70.77), Specificity (73.08), Sensitivity (61.54)	Lu *et al.* [38]
	-	364	-	2019/ UK	RPV: A Novel Prognostic Signature Discovered	Lu *et al.* [39]
	Unsupervised Hierarchical	469	N/A	2018/ Singapore & Malaysia	Accuracy (80.60 ± 0.5%), Sensitivity (81.40%), Specificity (76.30%)	Acharya *et al.* [40]
Pancreatic Neuroendocrine	Clustering	8422	23–90	2018 China	Accuracy (81.6% ± 1.9%), curve(0.87)	Song *et al.* [41]
Spinal Chordoma	Fuzzy Forest	265	-	2018 USA	5-year Survival (67.5%)	Karhade *et al.* [42]
	SVM, RF, DL		59(48–69)	-	-	-
	Boosted DT, SVM, ANN	-	N/A	-	-	-

Table 2. AI applied for cancer prognosis by the different researchers.

Methods	Number of Patients in the Study	Region/Year	Study Population	Results	Authors and Year
DCNN	17627	China, 2019	Both	Sensitivity (93.4%), CI (95%,89.6–96.1)	Li *et al.* [43]
CNN	203	China, 2019	Hospital	AUC (over 91%)	Zhu *et al.* [44]
Convolutional Autoencoder, Supervised Encoder FusionNet	374	Italy, 2019	Lymphoma and IDC Datasets	F-measure Score Improved (5.06%), Accuracy Improved (5.06%)	Nadia *et al.* [45]
CNN	Ensemble	India, 2019	TCGA	Accuracy (92.61%)	Tabibu *et al.* [46]
DCNN	2566	USA, 2018	Both	AUC(0.85 ± 0.05)	Samala *et al.* [47]
DCNN(inception v3)	137	USA, 2018	TCGA,NCI Genomic Data	AUC(0.733–0.856)	Coudray *et al.* [48]
Bayesian network	1034	Italy, 2018	Hospital	No conclusion	Wu *et al.* [49]
Decision Tree J48	436	Italy, 2018	Hospital	Accuracy (80%)	Yi *et al.* [50]
Inception v3 CNN	2032	USA, 2017	Both	AUC (over 91%)	Esteva *et al.* [51]
ANN	928	Germany, 2002	Hospital	Specificity Level (90%)	Stephan *et al.* [52]
Multivariate Cluster Analysis	98	Italy, 1999	Hospital	No reported conclusion	Lorenzo *et al.* [53]

Overall, researchers use AI in the area of cancer diagnosis and customised medicine for identifying the best care options for cancer patients as shown in Tables **1** and **2**. Although excellent results are coming, thorough research is still needed to further improve outcomes [54 - 57].

4. CHALLENGES FOR AI IN CANCER TREATMENT

However, precision, accuracy and efficiency of AI and machine learning have been established in the diagnosis and prognosis of various cancers; in certain contexts, this method aids in the early diagnosis of cancer-related lethal diseases and has resulted in reducing the reported mortality rates linked to multiple type of cancers . But there is still a long way to go. To ensure its application in cancer diagnosis and prognosis, AI faces certain hurdles to address [58].

Since images from medical imaging would not be used directly as input data, to maintain the precision and quality of the operation, it is necessary to retrieve and process features from the pictorial data by applying different mathematical models [59]. With the advancement of several AI-based technologies, medical specialists are in dire need to collaborate with machine experts.

One fear associated with depending on AI and ML is that the physician's value could decline when their efficiency would be superseded by AI [60, 61]. Privacy and data security assurances [62] are other crucial issues for the future of AI in medicine. In recent years, it has been noted that ML has facilitated medical experts to evaluate the enormous data.

Physicians, health, and science practitioners require a helping hand to encourage society with population increase and discoveries on various diseases. To set the optimum dose of chemo and radiotherapy for cancer patients and enhance their lifespan, researchers are trying to create ML. Dynamic non-linear associations may be controlled by AI (like chemotherapy and radiotherapy).

CONSENT FOR PUBLICATION

Not Applicable.

CONFLICT OF INTEREST

The author confirms that this chapter contents have no conflict of interest.

ACKNOWLEDGEMENT

Declared none.

REFERENCES

[1]   Simon S. Facts & Fig.s 2019: US Cancer Death Rate has Dropped 27% in 25 Years. Retrieved from: https://www.cancer.org/latest-news/facts-and-Fig.s-2019.html

[2]   Anees A. Applications of Artificial Intelligence in Cancer Diagnosis and Treatment 2019. Retrieved from: https://mesowatch.com/applications-of-artificial-intelligence-in-cancer-diagnosis-and-treatment/

[3]   Rebecca L. Cancer statistics. CA Cancer J Clin 2019; 69(1): 7-34.
[http://dx.doi.org/10.3322/caac.21551] [PMID: 30620402]

[4]   Obermeyer Z, Emanuel EJ. Predicting the future - big data, machine learning, and clinical medicine. N Engl J Med 2016; 375(13): 1216-9.
[http://dx.doi.org/10.1056/NEJMp1606181] [PMID: 27682033]

[5]   Hosny A, Parmar C, Quackenbush J, Schwartz LH, Aerts HJWL. Artificial intelligence in radiology. Nat Rev Cancer 2018; 18(8): 500-10.
[http://dx.doi.org/10.1038/s41568-018-0016-5] [PMID: 29777175]

[6]   Huang S, Yang J, Fong S, Zhao Q. Artificial intelligence in cancer diagnosis and prognosis: Opportunities and challenges. Cancer Lett 2020; 471: 61-71.

[http://dx.doi.org/10.1016/j.canlet.2019.12.007] [PMID: 31830558]

[7] Retrieved from. https://ourworldindata.org/canceron

[8] Retrieved from. https://www.technologynetworks.com/diagnostics/news/ai-for-lung-cancer-diagn ost ics-314929

[9] Retrieved from. https://transmitter.ieee.org/artificial-intelligence-is-now-detecting-breast-cancer-from-biopsy-images/

[10] Retrieved from. https://www.onartificialintelligence.com/articles/19416/prostrate-cancer-can-now-be-diagnosed-better-using-ai

[11] Yala A, Lehman C, Schuster T, Portnoi T, Barzilay R. A deep learning mammography-based model for improved breast cancer risk prediction. Radiology 2019; 292(1): 60-6.
[http://dx.doi.org/10.1148/radiol.2019182716] [PMID: 31063083]

[12] Retrieved from. https://www.europeanpharmaceuticalreview.com/news/36322/breakthrough-therap--designation-for-keytruda-in-advanced-colorectal-cancer/

[13] Hornbrook MC, Goshen R, Choman E, *et al.* Early colorectal cancer detected by machine learning model using gender, age, and complete blood count data. Dig Dis Sci 2017; 62(10): 2719-27.
[http://dx.doi.org/10.1007/s10620-017-4722-8] [PMID: 28836087]

[14] Xiao Z, Huang R, Ding Y, *et al.* A deep learning-based segmentation method for brain tumor in MR images. IEEE 6th International Conference on Computational Advances in Bio and Medical Sciences (ICCABS).
[http://dx.doi.org/10.1109/ICCABS.2016.7802771]

[15] Profiling the cancer genome to optimize the management of solid tumors. Retrieved from: https://www.sophiagenetics.com/hospitals/solutions/solutions/STS.html

[16] Dang YZ, Li X, Ma YX, *et al.* ^{18}F-FDG-PET/CT-guided intensity-modulated radiotherapy for 42 FIGO III/IV ovarian cancer: A retrospective study. Oncol Lett 2019; 17(1): 149-58.
[PMID: 30655750]

[17] Gao HX, Huang SG, Du JF, *et al.* J.F. Du, X.C. Zhang, N. Jiang, W.X. Kang, J. Mao, Q. Zhao, Comparison of prognostic indices in NSCLC patients with brain metastases after radiosurgery. Int J Biol Sci 2018; 14(14): 2065-72.
[http://dx.doi.org/10.7150/ijbs.28608] [PMID: 30585269]

[18] Enshaei A, Robson CN, Edmondson RJ. Robson, R.J. Edmondson, Artificial intelligence systems as prognostic and predictive tools in ovarian cancer. Ann Surg Oncol 2015; 22(12): 3970-5.
[http://dx.doi.org/10.1245/s10434-015-4475-6] [PMID: 25752894]

[19] S.H. Khan, U, J.P. Choi, *et al.* wFDT weighted fuzzy decision trees for prognosis of breast cancer survivability. Proceedings of the 7th Australasian Data Mining Conference, Australian Computer Society. 141-52.

[20] Sun D, Wang M, Li A. A multimodal deep neural network for human breast cancer prognosis prediction by integrating multi-dimensional data. IEEE/ACM Trans Comput Biol Bioinformatics 2018; 16(3): 841-50.
[http://dx.doi.org/10.1109/TCBB.2018.2806438] [PMID: 29994639]

[21] Park K, Ali A, Kim D, An Y, Kim M, Shin H. Robust predictive model for evaluating breast cancer survivability. Eng Appl Artif Intell 2013; 26: 2194-205.
[http://dx.doi.org/10.1016/j.engappai.2013.06.013]

[22] Delen D, Walker G, Kadam A. Predicting breast cancer survivability: a comparison of three data mining methods. Artif Intell Med 2005; 34(2): 113-27.
[http://dx.doi.org/10.1016/j.artmed.2004.07.002] [PMID: 15894176]

[23] Lu H, Wang H, Yoon SW. A dynamic gradient boosting machine using genetic optimizer for practical breast cancer prognosis. Expert Syst Appl 2019; 116: 340-50.

[http://dx.doi.org/10.1016/j.eswa.2018.08.040]

[24]   Tian DW, Wu ZL, Jiang LM, Gao J, Wu CL, Hu HL. Neural precursor cell expressed, developmentally downregulated 8 promotes tumor progression and predicts poor prognosis of patients with bladder cancer. Cancer Sci 2019; 110(1): 458-67.
[http://dx.doi.org/10.1111/cas.13865] [PMID: 30407690]

[25]   Hasnain Z, Mason J, Gill K, *et al.* Machine learning models for predicting post-cystectomy recurrence and survival in bladder cancer patients. PLoS One 2019; 14(2): e0210976.
[http://dx.doi.org/10.1371/journal.pone.0210976] [PMID: 30785915]

[26]   Bottaci L, Drew PJ, Hartley JE, *et al.* Artificial neural networks applied to outcome prediction for colorectal cancer patients in separate institutions. Lancet 1997; 350(9076): 469-72.
[http://dx.doi.org/10.1016/S0140-6736(96)11196-X] [PMID: 9274582]

[27]   Wang Y, Wang D, Ye X, Wang Y, Yin Y, Jin Y. A tree ensemble-based two-stage model for advanced-stage colorectal cancer survival prediction. Inf Sci 2019; 474: 106-24.
[http://dx.doi.org/10.1016/j.ins.2018.09.046]

[28]   Bychkov D, Linder N, Turkki R, *et al.* Deep learning based tissue analysis predicts outcome in colorectal cancer. Sci Rep 2018; 8(1): 3395.
[http://dx.doi.org/10.1038/s41598-018-21758-3] [PMID: 29467373]

[29]   Biglarian A, Hajizadeh E, Kazemnejad A, Zali M. Application of artificial neural network in predicting the survival rate of gastric cancer patients. Iran J Public Health 2011; 40(2): 80-6.
[PMID: 23113076]

[30]   Zhu L, Luo W, Su M, *et al.* Comparison between artificial neural network and Cox regression model in predicting the survival rate of gastric cancer patients. Biomed Rep 2013; 1(5): 757-60.
[http://dx.doi.org/10.3892/br.2013.140] [PMID: 24649024]

[31]   Lu CF, Hsu FT, Hsieh KL, *et al.* Machine learning-based radiomics for molecular subtyping of gliomas. Clin Cancer Res 2018; 24(18): 4429-36.
[http://dx.doi.org/10.1158/1078-0432.CCR-17-3445] [PMID: 29789422]

[32]   Papp L, Pötsch N, Grahovac M, *et al.* Glioma survival prediction with combined analysis of *in vivo* (11)C-met PET features, *ex vivo* features, and patient features by supervised machine learning. J Nucl Med 2018; 59(6): 892-9.
[http://dx.doi.org/10.2967/jnumed.117.202267] [PMID: 29175980]

[33]   Janssen SJ, van der Heijden AS, van Dijke M, *et al.* Marshall urist young investigator award: prognostication in patients with long bone metastases: does a boosting algorithm improve survival estimates? Clin. Orthop Relat Res 2015; 473(2015): 3112-21.

[34]   Lynch CM, Abdollahi B, Fuqua JD, *et al.* Prediction of lung cancer patient survival *via* supervised machine learning classification techniques. Int J Med Inform 2017; 108: 1-8.
[http://dx.doi.org/10.1016/j.ijmedinf.2017.09.013] [PMID: 29132615]

[35]   Sepehri S, Upadhaya T, Desseroit M-C, Visvikis D, Le Rest CC, Hatt M. Comparison of machine learning algorithms for building prognostic models in non-small cell lung cancer using clinical and radiomics features from 18F-FDG PET/CT images. J Nucl Med 2018; 59: 328-8.

[36]   Yu KH, Zhang C, Berry GJ, *et al.* Predicting non-small cell lung cancer prognosis by fully automated microscopic pathology image features. Nat Commun 2016; 7: 12474.
[http://dx.doi.org/10.1038/ncomms12474] [PMID: 27527408]

[37]   Lu C, Lewis JS Jr, Dupont WD, Plummer WD Jr, Janowczyk A, Madabhushi A. An oral cavity squamous cell carcinoma quantitative histomorphometric-based image classifier of nuclear morphology can risk stratify patients for disease-specific survival. Mod Pathol 2017; 30(12): 1655-65.
[http://dx.doi.org/10.1038/modpathol.2017.98] [PMID: 28776575]

[38]   Lu H, Arshad M, Thornton A, *et al.* A mathematical-descriptor of tumor-mesoscopic-structure from computed-tomography images annotates prognostic- and molecular-phenotypes of epithelial ovarian

cancer. Nat Commun 2019; 10(1): 764.
[http://dx.doi.org/10.1038/s41467-019-08718-9] [PMID: 30770825]

[39]   Acharya UR, Akter A, Chowriappa P, *et al.* Use of nonlinear features for automated characterization of suspicious ovarian tumors using ultrasound images in fuzzy forest framework. Int J Fuzzy Syst 2018; 20.
[http://dx.doi.org/10.1007/s40815-018-0456-9]

[40]   Song Y, Gao S, Tan W, Qiu Z, Zhou H, Zhao Y. Multiple machine learnings revealed similar predictive accuracy for prognosis of pnets from the surveillance, epidemiology, and end result database. J Cancer 2018; 9(21): 3971-8.
[http://dx.doi.org/10.7150/jca.26649] [PMID: 30410601]

[41]   Karhade AV, Thio Q, Ogink P, *et al.* Development of machine learning algorithms for prediction of 5-year spinal chordoma survival. World Neurosurg 2018; 119: e842-7.
[http://dx.doi.org/10.1016/j.wneu.2018.07.276] [PMID: 30096498]

[42]   Li X, Zhang S, Zhang Q, *et al.* Diagnosis of thyroid cancer using deep convolutional neural network models applied to sonographic images: a retrospective, multicohort, diagnostic study. Lancet Oncol 2019; 20(2): 193-201.
[http://dx.doi.org/10.1016/S1470-2045(18)30762-9] [PMID: 30583848]

[43]   Zhu Y, Wang QC, Xu MD, *et al.* Application of convolutional neural network in the diagnosis of the invasion depth of gastric cancer based on conventional endoscopy. Gastrointest Endosc 2009; 89(4): 806-815.e1.
[http://dx.doi.org/10.1016/j.gie.2018.11.011]

[44]   Brancati N, De Pietro G, Frucci M, Riccio D. A deep learning approach for breast invasive ductal carcinoma detection and lymphoma multi-classification in histological images. IEEE Access 2019; 7: 44709-20.
[http://dx.doi.org/10.1109/ACCESS.2019.2908724]

[45]   Tabibu S, Vinod PK, Jawahar CV. A Deep Learning Approach for Pan-Renal Cell Carcinoma Classification and Survival Prediction from Histopathology Images. 2019.

[46]   Samala RK, Heang-Ping Chan , Hadjiiski L, Helvie MA, Richter CD, Cha KH. Breast cancer diagnosis in digital breast tomosynthesis: effects of training sample size on multi-stage transfer learning using deep neural nets. IEEE Trans Med Imaging 2019; 38(3): 686-96.
[http://dx.doi.org/10.1109/TMI.2018.2870343] [PMID: 31622238]

[47]   Coudray N, Ocampo PS, Sakellaropoulos T, *et al.* Classification and mutation prediction from non-small cell lung cancer histopathology images using deep learning. Nat Med 2018; 24(10): 1559-67.
[http://dx.doi.org/10.1038/s41591-018-0177-5] [PMID: 30224757]

[48]   Wu Y, Lin L, Shen Y, Wu H. Comparison between PD-1/PD-L1 inhibitors (nivolumab, pembrolizumab, and atezolizumab) in pretreated NSCLC patients: Evidence from a Bayesian network model. Int J Cancer 2018; 143(11): 3038-40.
[http://dx.doi.org/10.1002/ijc.31733] [PMID: 29987914]

[49]   Yi X, Guan X, Chen C, *et al.* Adrenal incidentaloma: machine learning-based quantitative texture analysis of unenhanced CT can effectively differentiate sPHEO from lipid-poor adrenal adenoma. J Cancer 2018; 9(19): 3577-82.
[http://dx.doi.org/10.7150/jca.26356] [PMID: 30310515]

[50]   Haenssle HA, Fink C, Schneiderbauer R, *et al.* I. Reader study level, I.I.G. level, Man against machine: diagnostic performance of a deep learning convolutional neural network for dermoscopic melanoma recognition in comparison to 58 dermatologists. Ann Oncol 2018; 29: 1836-42.
[http://dx.doi.org/10.1093/annonc/mdy166] [PMID: 29846502]

[51]   Esteva A, Kuprel B, Novoa RA, *et al.* Dermatologist-level classification of skin cancer with deep neural networks. Nature 2017; 542(7639): 115-8.
[http://dx.doi.org/10.1038/nature21056] [PMID: 28117445]

[52]   Stephan C, Jung K, Cammann H, *et al.* An artificial neural network considerably improves the diagnostic power of percent free prostate-specific antigen in prostate cancer diagnosis: results of a 5-year investigation. Int J Cancer 2002; 99(3): 466-73.
[http://dx.doi.org/10.1002/ijc.10370] [PMID: 11992419]

[53]   Leoncini L, Cossu A, Megha T, *et al.* Expression of p34(cdc2) and cyclins A and B compared to other proliferative features of non-Hodgkin's lymphomas: a multivariate cluster analysis. Int J Cancer 1999; 83(2): 203-9.
[http://dx.doi.org/10.1002/(SICI)1097-0215(19991008)83:2<203::AID-IJC10>3.0.CO;2-0]   [PMID: 10471528]

[54]   Retrieved From: IBM and Pfizer to Accelerate Immuno-oncology Research with Watson for Drug Discovery. https://www.pfizer.com/news/press-release/press-release-detail/ibm_and_pfizer_to_accele rate_immuno_oncology_research_with_watson_for_drug_discovery.

[55]   Retrieved from: National Cancer Institute, "Cancer Statistics." Accessed 18 November 2016. Available at http://ibm.biz/Bdsqw9

[56]   Van Noorden R. Scientists may be reaching a peak in reading habits http://ibm.biz/BdrAjS2014.
[http://dx.doi.org/10.1038/nature.2014.14658]

[57]   Thurtle DR, Greenberg DC, Lee LS, Huang HH, Pharoah PD, Gnanapragasam VJ. Individual prognosis at diagnosis in nonmetastatic prostate cancer: Development and external validation of the PREDICT Prostate multivariable model. PLoS Med 2019; 16(3): e1002758.
[http://dx.doi.org/10.1371/journal.pmed.1002758] [PMID: 30860997]

[58]   Feng H, Gu ZY, Li Q, Liu QH, Yang XY, Zhang JJ. Identification of significant genes with poor prognosis in ovarian cancer *via* bioinformatical analysis. J Ovarian Res 2019; 12(1): 35.
[http://dx.doi.org/10.1186/s13048-019-0508-2] [PMID: 31010415]

[59]   Qian D, Liu H, Wang X, *et al.* Potentially functional genetic variants in the complement-related immunity gene-set are associated with non-small cell lung cancer survival. Int J Cancer 2019; 144(8): 1867-76.
[http://dx.doi.org/10.1002/ijc.31896] [PMID: 30259978]

[60]   Cabitza F, Rasoini R, Gensini GF. Unintended consequences of machine learning in medicine. JAMA 2017; 318(6): 517-8.
[http://dx.doi.org/10.1001/jama.2017.7797] [PMID: 28727867]

[61]   Topol EJ. High-performance medicine: the convergence of human and artificial intelligence. Nat Med 2019; 25(1): 44-56.
[http://dx.doi.org/10.1038/s41591-018-0300-7] [PMID: 30617339]

[62]   Fröhlich H, Balling R, Beerenwinkel N, *et al.* From hype to reality: data science enabling personalized medicine. BMC Med 2018; 16(1): 150.
[http://dx.doi.org/10.1186/s12916-018-1122-7] [PMID: 30145981]

CHAPTER 2

Alternative or Auxiliary: Artificial Intelligence Accelerates the Development and Transformation of the Medical Care

Jie Yang[1,2,*], **Quanyi Hu**[1], **Rui Tang**[3], **Han Wang**[4,5], **Kairong Duan**[1,6], **Feng Wu**[5] and **Simon Fong**[1,5]

[1] *Department of Computer and Information Science, University of Macau, Macau, China*

[2] *Chongqing Industry & Trade Polytechnic, Chongqing, China*

[3] *Department of Management Science and Information System, Faculty of Management and Economics, Kunming University of Science and Technology, Kunming, China*

[4] *Faculty of Data Science, City University of Macau, Taipa, Macao, China*

[5] *Zhuhai Institutes of Advanced Technology of the Chinese Academy of Sciences, China*

[6] *Department of Electrical Engineering and Computer Sciences, University of California, Berkeley, CA, USA*

Abstract: The application of artificial intelligence has been in full swing in all walks of life, especially in the medical field, which has been favored and achieved remarkable results. This paper explores its application and development prospects by analyzing the fundamental principle of AI and its application in the medical-relevant industry and discusses its role in the medical field, which is more an aid than a substitute. Meanwhile, the application of AI in medical care is relatively lagging behind and has a lot of room for development compared with other fields. AI technology should be applied to the medical field in a targeted manner to deal with bottlenecks and exert greater potential and value.

Keywords: Artificial intelligence, Big data, Deep learning, Machine learning, Medical care.

1. INTRODUCTION

With the emergence of big data and the improvement of people's familiarity with big data, various fields of technological development are constantly innovating,

* **Corresponding author Jie Yang:** Department of Computer and Information Science, University of Macau; Chongqing Industry & Trade Polytechnic, Chongqing, China; Tel: 86 02372802117, Fax: 86 02372802117; E-mail: jie.yang@ieee.org

including artificial intelligence (AI) development, which also means that human society is featured with the intelligence era. With the rapid development of AI, various industries are changing their models and adapting to the development of the times [33 - 38], including medical care and public health industry, where AI has played an important role.

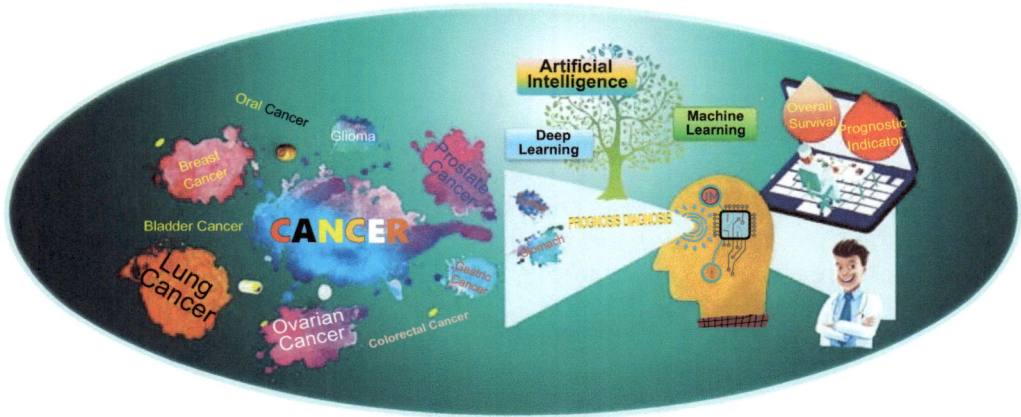

Fig. (1). Schematic diagram of AI diagnosis and prediction of cancer.

2. ABOUT ARTIFICIAL INTELLIGENCE

Artificial intelligence is a new technology that researches and develops theories, methods, technologies, and application systems for simulating and extending human intelligence. It includes machine learning and deep learning. Its structure is similar to a pyramid structure: the upper layer is an algorithm, the middle is the chip, the third layer is a variety of hardware and software platforms, and the bottom is the application [1]. Research in the field of AI is basically the formal use of the term "artificial intelligence" at a conference held at Dartmouth University in 1956, marking the beginning of AI [2]. In the following decades, people conducted extensive research on AI. As a branch of computer science, it attempted to produce a new intelligent machine that responded to the human brain by mining the essence of intelligence. Application areas of technology include robotics, image recognition, language recognition, natural language processing, data mining, pattern recognition, and expert systems [3 - 6].

3. APPLICATION STATUS AND DEVELOPMENT PROSPECTS IN THE MEDICAL INDUSTRY

The characteristics of AI, such as service robot, remote video diagnosis, and advanced CT technology, will significantly fulfill the "human replace innovation" (HRI) with many repetitive, regular, and dangerous tasks, for example, the diagnosis and prognosis of AI in cancer medicine have been comparable to experienced experts.

Fig. **(1)** shows a schematic diagram of AI in the application of diagnosis and prediction of cancer. By training with large data and samples, AI models can achieve a more realistic effect, improve the efficiency of medical testing in cancer diagnosis and shorten the diagnosis and recovery period of patients. However, AI will not change the essence of the medical profession nor replace the doctor's diagnosis and treatment. For example, although the speed and accuracy of machine readings exceed that of doctors [7], the treatment plan provided is single, and it is difficult to combine the individual conditions of patients to provide the best treatment plan that meets the individual needs of patients. In short, the goal of exploring the application of AI in the medical field is to enhance the precision of the diagnosis, assist and promote the medical industry in terms of human enhancing innovation (HEI), rather than relying on equipment and machines to replace the medical profession [8].

3.1. Current Status of the Application of AI

In 2019, the Chinese Academy of Sciences published its core magazine "the Internet Weekly" and listed the TOP 100 AI cases, " [9], 17 of which are directly relevant to the application of AI in the medical and public health industry, as shown in Table **1**. This shows that the application of AI in medical treatment has extensive and huge development prospects. The following is a brief introduction to several typical fields of AI in the medical industry.

3.1.1. Intelligent Services in the Ageing Society

The United Nations' dataset "World Population Prospects: 2019 Revision" showed that in 2018, the global population of 65 years or older has unprecedentedly exceeded the number of people under five. By 2050, 1 out of 6 in the world will be over 65 years old (16%). This number will be 11 (9%) in 2019. In addition, the population aged 80 or over is expected to triple, from 143 million in 2019 to 426 million in 2050 [10]. The breakthrough of AI technology has created a smart pension service industry with robots and intelligent technology as the core and has become the most potential to achieve the goal of a pension service system based on community, medical institution supplement, and medical care. The preferred solution of this program, the application of intelligent robots in elderly care, mainly completes the following work.

Table 1. The "2019 Artificial Intelligence Cases TOP100" from "Internet Weekly" published by the director of the Chinese Academy of Sciences and hosted by the Science Press, 17 of which are the application of AI in medical treatment, accounting for 17%.

No.	Procurement	Tender	Case
1	Health Commission of Ningbo	YiduCloud	Ningbo Comprehensive Surveillance and Service Platform
2	Tianjin Diabetes Screen and Transfer Platform	VoxelCloud	VoxelCloudRetina Disease Screening
3	Guangzhou Baiyun Airport	CloudWalk	AI Epidemic Prevention and Detection
4	Shanghai Jiaotong University	Ping An Healthcare & Technology Company	One Minute Doctor by Ping And Good Doctor
5	First Affiliated Hospital of Kunming Medical University	HiAR	AR/5 COVID-19 3D Digital Internet-based Remote Consultation System
6	The Fifth Affiliated Hospital of Sun Yat-Sen University	Huiyi Huiying	Dr. Turing COVID-19 AI Screening System
7	China-Japan Friendship Hospital	Deepwise	Computer Aided Diagnosis for Micro Pulmonary Nodules
8	Peking University Shougang Hospital,Wuhan Huoshenshan Hospital, Beijing Haidian Hospital, Zhengzhou Qiboshan Hospital	Cheetah Mobile	AI Robot Medical Solution for COVID-19
9	Renji Hospital,School of Medicine, Shanghai Jiaotong University	Kyee Group	Mobile Medical Solution
10	Sichuan Province People's Hospital	PereDoc	AI Smart Medical Integral Solution
11	Obstetrics & Gynecology Hospital of Fudan University	Wondersgroup	AI Clinical Aided Solution for Advanced Aged Pregnancy
12	Changsha Public Security Bureau	Centrin Ciyun	NLP-based Medical Corpus Recognition Application
13	Linyi Shandong Energy Mining Group Co. Ltd	Luculent	AI-enabled Equipment Management and Diagnose Platform
14	Central Hospital of Qinghe County	Xueyang Technology	AI Early Warning Solution for Myocardial Infarction and Apoplexy
15	Haidian Administrative Service Hall, Haidian Mudanyuan Subway Station	Megvii	AI-enabled Temperature Screening Solution

(Table 1) cont.....

No.	Procurement	Tender	Case
16	Wuhan Union Hospital,Party School Hospital and Isolation Spot	Keenon	Peanut Robot
17	Wuhou District Government, Chengdu	Geotmt	Robot for COVID-19 Prevention

1. Assisting the elderly to complete daily tasks: The nursing robot RQEAR (shaped like a panda face) developed in Japan in 2015 is used to help people with reduced mobility. It can pick up, put down or help people stand with gentle movements. Another nursing robot developed by Panasonic Corporation can be multi-functional, such as a bed and electric wheelchair, to complete the tasks of multiple caregivers alone [11].

2. Monitoring the behavior and health status of the elderly: The German Lerks Robotics Institute provides a nursing robot for the elderly, which can detect the health status of the elderly, help them take medicine from another room, and make medication records for the elderly [12]. The SAM janitor robot of the United States LUVOZO company can provide frequent long-term rounds of rounds and non-pharmaceutical care services for the elderly at home with automatic navigation, remote monitoring, and anti-tumbling detection systems [13].

3. Providing companionship: Israel's Intuition Robotics developed ElliQ, a "sidekick for happier aging." Companion robots with AI can talk to patients, remind them to take drugs, and lead them to perform light physical activities to improve physical and mental health. ElliQ can be integrated with the various message and social media platforms, enabling users to send and receive text and pictures without using a mobile phone. The nursing robot "Zola" has been introduced in nursing homes in Australia. The robot can fulfill multiple entertainment purposes such as sports, dance, read books, tell jokes, and actual communication with the elderly based on speech recognition technology [14].

4. Comprehensive solution: The researchers from the IBM elderly care solution seek to provide a kind of relief for the elderly, which comes from having a private nurse. It involves motion sensors in corridors, flush detectors in toilets, and bed sensors monitoring sleep quality. Any major deviation from the normal activity pattern can send an automatic alarm to an authorized nurse or doctor. The system can also track the health indicators of the elderly and actively foresee risks. By using machine learning algorithms to analyze historical data, researchers can also discover unknown and predicted relationships such as the relationship between daily living habits and unusual sleeping habits or the relationship between the irregular nighttime toilet and the risk of tumbling. Overall, the system seeks to identify early warning signals that may require additional attention.

The UNESCO World Scientific Knowledge and Technology Ethics Committee (COMEST) released a report expressing concerns about the application of AI in aging care technology. The report pointed out that protecting human dignity and privacy is also applicable to the field of unknown intelligent robots [13]. Related ethical risks involve safety, privacy, integrity, dignity, and autonomy. For example, the patient may refuse to take medicines for reasonable reasons if an elderly care robot reminds a patient to take medicine, and the robot needs to know what to do at this time. It is still one of the difficulties and challenges in the current AI technology, in addition, the robot "believes" that it is reasonable to prevent the elderly from gaining weight and therefore prohibit them from eating high-calorie foods. There may also be another situation where the guardian's remote control robot restrains the elderly, resulting in potential hidden dangers in morality and law. At this stage, the development of elderly care robot products mainly focuses on the application of AI technology to improve the basic capabilities of home machine partners. The application of elderly care robots, in the future, will focus on improving the development of higher-end intelligent services such as the quality of life, personalized companionship, health monitoring, and disease treatment of the elderly.

3.1.2. Smart Ward

Traditional wards are only a venue for medical staff to provide medical services to patients. The workload of medical staff is high, and sometimes, the hospitalization experience of patients is also poor due to the shortage of medical resources. In order to alleviate this stressful pressure, the Smart Ward Information System ("SWIS"), through the Internet (Internet), Internet of Things (IoT), cloud computing and other technologies, create digital-AI-based smart wards. The United States and the United Kingdom have fully implemented the practice of AI associated with medical care. Thomas Jefferson University Hospital, head-quartered in Philadelphia, launched a smart ward supported by IBM Watson Internet of Things in 2016. Through IBM's cognitive computing and natural language performance, patients can possess their passwords during hospitalization, operate lights, shutters, sounds, *etc.*, through indoor speakers to adjust light, adjust room temperature, and turn on music to meet the patient's needs for the ward environment. Meanwhile, the patient can obtain some kind of information and action assistance that he wants to know through dialogue with the system. In addition, the platform can assist medical staff in carrying out interactive dialogues with patients, and record and store the dialogue contents for future medical examinations. The intelligent ward aims to improve the patient's hospitalization experience and to reduce the workload of medical staff through profound, flexible, and personalized reactive care. Alder Hey Children's Hospital in Liverpool, UK, recently developed a doctor-patient communication application software in cooperation with the British Science and Technology Commission and conducted exercises in the ward. The children and their families are asked to provide basic information when entering the hospital, including food allergy, favorite games and movies favorite, colors, and bedroom environment. The family members of the children are also asked questions about medical procedures, anesthesia, and surgery history. The information is used to develop intelligent application software through an interactive platform. The communication link between the child and his family before admission helps the family of the child understand the necessary information before admission, making the entire admission process smoother and time-saving [15]. The main feature of SWIS is that the patient is the center, and the sickbed is the platform, with patient health data management as the mainline, connecting the medical institution HIS system and various management subsystems through the SWIS system. It also closely connects patients, medical staff, and medical monitoring equipment through multiple networks, with low-cost and high-efficiency construction of a patient-centric health care platform, also achieves the patient's perception and operability and improves the patient's medical experience during hospitalization, which reduce the intensity of workload and operational costs, and improve the efficiency of medical care.

3.1.3. Hazard Warning Identification

Most diseases are preventable, but brain diseases are usually not easy to detect in the early stage, such a disease is not discovered until the deterioration of the patient's health status. Although doctors can use tools to assist in disease prediction, the complexity of the human body and the diversity of diseases can affect the accuracy of prediction. The combination of AI technology and medical health wearable devices can realize disease risk prediction and actual intervention. Risk prediction includes an early warning of personal health status and monitoring of public health events such as epidemics, and intervention mainly refers to personalized health management and consulting services for different patients. The machine analyzes, integrates, and develops the data with fast and accurate judgment on the identification of upsetting signals in various diseases and their treatment, which can avoid some serious consequences or complications. Alzheimer's can be indentified in the early stages, but the detection is relatively difficult. The sooner the disease is detected, the better the chance for patients to seek early treatment and reduce the aftermath of the disease. The clinical diagnosis of Alzheimer's requires comprehensive judgment by means of neuropsychological tests, hematological, structural, or functional imaging examinations, and electroencephalograms. The difficulty in diagnosis and treatment of Alzheimer's lies in the non-specificity of symptoms and test indicators, and it is difficult to achieve early diagnosis. By inputting three different types of data, such as MRI, EEG, and scale, companies such as Yasen Technology comprehensively use machine training, statistical analysis, and deep learning methods to find out whether the patient is getting illness and the relationship between the input information. For the AI used in the diagnosis of Alzheimer's, it is not only the recognition of medical images in the traditional sense of deep learning, but on this basis, it aims to find out the relationship between multiple information sources and based on these data, trains a multimodal neural network model to predict the likelihood of developing Alzheimer' and the stage of the disease's development two or three years in advance [16].

Sugar retinopathy is retinopathy caused by diabetes. Statistically, about 500 million people in China are pre-diabetic, about 110 million people with diabetes, and about 30 million people with diabetic retinopathy. Fundus screening for diabetic patients is of great significance because early diagnosis of patients with sugar retinopathy is usually difficult, and the symptoms are not obvious. Only after an early screening of the fundus, timely detection of sugar retinopathy and early intervention can effectively resist the disease. Compared with the diagnosis of other diseases that need to be combined with clinical information, the examination in the field of diabetic retinopathy fundus with AI has higher operability because only the examination of the eye image has higher diagnostic value. For lesions such as exudation or bleeding, the AI system can also ensure higher accuracy. In addition, researchers are further studying how to use social media to collect information about mental health to establish a population model that can be used by social policy decision-makers as well as a warning based on cross-applied keywords learned by the system.

3.1.4. Assistance in Disease Diagnosis

In the mid-1980s, Judea Pearl's formalism made Bayesian networks popular on computers. Since then, AI has begun to explore and implement clinical diagnosis problems [17, 32]. With the rise of neural network technology in medical expert systems, the application of AI in medical diagnosis has shown a primary improvement. In terms of medical image and voice recognition, the "artificial momentum substrate" developed by the Mitsubishi Electromechanical Research Institute in Japan can quickly and accurately identify a large number of medical image information [18]. In terms of medical diagnosis, Topalovic and others have developed a machine learning framework that simulates the human brain's cognition to analyze complex medical data, automatically interprets pneumonia function tests and computed tomography results, and thereby diagnoses most common obstructive lung diseases; for example, chronic obstructive pulmonary disease (COPD), asthma, interstitial lung disease, *etc.*, for which, the general accuracy rate is 68% [19]. The successful application of this technology benefits from machine learning; it has a higher speed and a wider space, which can help doctors provide faster and highly accurate diagnoses [20].

3.1.5. Assistance in Drug Development and Disease Treatment

AI is restructuring the process of new drug research and development, greatly improving the efficiency of drug manufacturing. Traditional drug research and development requires a lot of time and money. It takes an average of $ 1 billion and about 10 years for a pharmaceutical company to successfully develop a new drug. Drug development needs to go through the stages of target screening, drug mining, clinical trials, and drug optimization. At present, Chinese pharmaceutical companies are deploying the field of AI, mainly in the stage of new drug production and clinical trials; for example, target screening, where the target refers to the binding site of drugs and biological macromolecules in the body, usually involving receptors, enzymes, ion channels, transporters, immune system, genes, *etc*. The key to the research and development of modern new drugs is to find, determine and prepare drug screening molecular drug targets, in which the traditional method is to cross-match the existing drugs on the market with more than 10,000 targets in the human body to find new and effective binding points. AI technology is expected to improve this process. AI can find available information from massive medical literature, papers, patents, clinical trial information, and other unstructured data and extract biological knowledge to make biochemical predictions. It is predicted that this method is expected to reduce the time and cost of drug development by approximately 50%.

Drug mining can also be termed as lead compound screening. It is based on a combination experiment of millions of small molecule compounds accumulated in the pharmaceutical industry to find compounds with a certain biological activity and chemical structure for further structural transformation and modification. There are two options for the application of AI technology in this process. One is to develop virtual screening technology to replace the high-throughput screening, and the other is to apply image recognition technology to optimize the high-throughput screening process. Using image recognition technology, we can evaluate the characteristics and effects of different disease cell models after administration and predict effective drug candidates. According to statistics, 90% of clinical trials failed to recruit a sufficient number and quality of patients in a timely manner. The use of AI to analyze the patient's medical records can more accurately dig into the target patient and improve the efficiency of recruiting patients.

In addition, although AI can not replace doctors' diagnosis and treatment, its auxiliary role for disease treatment is also not to be underestimated. AI plays a role in monitoring, compliance, and identification of side effects in the treatment process, ensuring the optimal effect and minimum risk of treatment. In a recent study using AI to reduce the risk of non-compliance in anticoagulation patients, researchers equipped mobile medical devices for patients participating in anticoagulation therapy, installed health risk assessment and behavioral accountability applications, and adopted the algorithm to determine the intake of oral drugs according to the patient's situation. The application provides drug reminders and dose instructions and triggers a delayed dose notification within one hour before the end of the dose window. The real-time data is encrypted and transmitted to the network-based dashboard for analysis. If the medicine is missed or delayed, or the patient does not take medicine correctly, the clinic staff will receive an automatic reminder by SMS or email. The use of this application helps to improve patient compliance and reduce side effects and harm caused by incorrect drug dosage [21 - 23].

3.1.6. Gene Sequencing

Gene sequencing is a new type of gene detection technology. It analyzes and determines gene sequences and can be used in clinical genetic disease diagnosis, prenatal screening, tumor prediction and treatment, and other fields. A single human genome has 3 billion base pairs and encodes approximately 23,000 genes containing functionality. Genetic testing is to mine valid information from massive data by decoding. At present, the operation level of high-throughput sequencing technology is mainly decoding and recording, and it is difficult to realize gene interpretation, so the sufficient information obtained from the gene sequence is very limited. The intervention of AI technology can improve the current technical obstacles. By establishing an initial mathematical model, the whole genome sequence and RNA sequence of a healthy person are imported into the model for training, and the model learns the RNA shear pattern of the healthy person. Afterward the trained model is modified by other molecular biology methods, and finally, the accuracy of the model is checked against the case data. Recently, IBM Watson, domestic leading companies such as Huada Gene, Boao Bio, and Jinyu, have all started their own AI layout. Taking Jinyu inspection as an example, the comprehensive inspection and detection technology platform to set up a disease-oriented testing center integrates new-generation information technologies such as biotechnology and AI to provide professional clinical testing services for the majority of patients. The genomic testing center of JinYu Testing incorporates whole-genome scanning, fluorescence *in situ* hybridization, cytogenetics, and traditional PCR information platform, and utilizes the high-throughput sequencing technology (HTS), the most revolutionary new technology in the field of gene sequencing, for clinical high-throughput, large-scale, automated and comprehensive genetic testing services. At the same time, Jinyu Inspection relies on massive medical test sample data covering more than 90% of the country 's population, serving more than 21,000 medical institutions annually, and over 40 million annual specimens covering different regions, different ethnic groups, and different age levels of the country. The "Precision Medical" Inspection and Testing Big Data Research Institute with Guangzhou characteristics was established.

3.2. Development Prospects of AI

Huang and Yang *et al.* [24] conducted a literature survey on the application of AI in cancer diagnosis and prognosis. Most of these papers contain keywords such as "machine learning," "deep learning," "AI" and "prognosis," discussing how AI can help in cancer diagnosis and prognosis, especially in terms of its unprecedented accuracy, which is even higher than the accuracy of general statistical applications in oncology. AI has expertise in cancer management and assisted decision support, which makes AI technology more of an auxiliary diagnosis and treatment rather than a substitute for doctors to participate in medical tasks.

3.2.1. Cancer Management: The Combination of Tumor Organic Chips and AI

Cancer is the second leading cause of death in the world. The number of deaths caused by cancer is about 13 million each year. It is estimated that there will be 22 million new cancer patients globally by 2030 [1, 25]. The treatment of cancer has always been a difficult problem in medicine. Chemotherapy is the main treatment method for cancer, but the side effects of chemotherapy are large, and the tumor is not necessarily sensitive to chemotherapy drugs. This treatment also has great limitations. Scientists from the University of Surrey and other institutions have developed a new AI system (AI) through research, which is expected to predict the symptoms and severity of the disease in cancer patients throughout the treatment process. The researchers described in detail how the two machine learning models they developed accurately predicted the severity of the three disease symptoms faced by cancer patients. These three symptoms include depression, anxiety, and sleep disorders, which are related to the quality of life of cancer patients. The apparent decline is directly related. The results of the study show that the symptoms actually reported by the patients are very close to the symptoms predicted by the machine learning method. Scientists have the opportunity to use machine-learning technology to modify the quality of life of cancer patients, which can help patients develop strategies to manage their symptoms and improve their quality of life [26]. Researchers are very pleased to use machine learning technology and AI technology to develop a series of strategies to bring certain help to the disease management of cancer patients (Fig. **2**). The team led by Professor Kamdar, deputy director of the Massachusetts General Hospital palliative care department, used a smartphone application powered by AI to monitor and control the pain of advanced cancer patients. The preliminary results of the study were published on PCOS on November 16, 2018. The latest research results were published on ASCO this time. The data shows that using the ePAL (Partners Health Care Pivot Labs) application, it reduces the pain of solid tumor cancer patients by 20% and reduces the pain-related hospitalization rate by 69%. The functions of ePAL include pain tracking, obstacle recognition, intervention, daily customized AI missionary information, an educational library, and physical and mental therapy [27]. "Nature" released an important study on cancer diagnosis. Scientists from the University of California, San Diego (UCSD), trained AI to identify clues from microorganisms in the blood, not only to identify cancer but also to distinguish between different types of cancer.

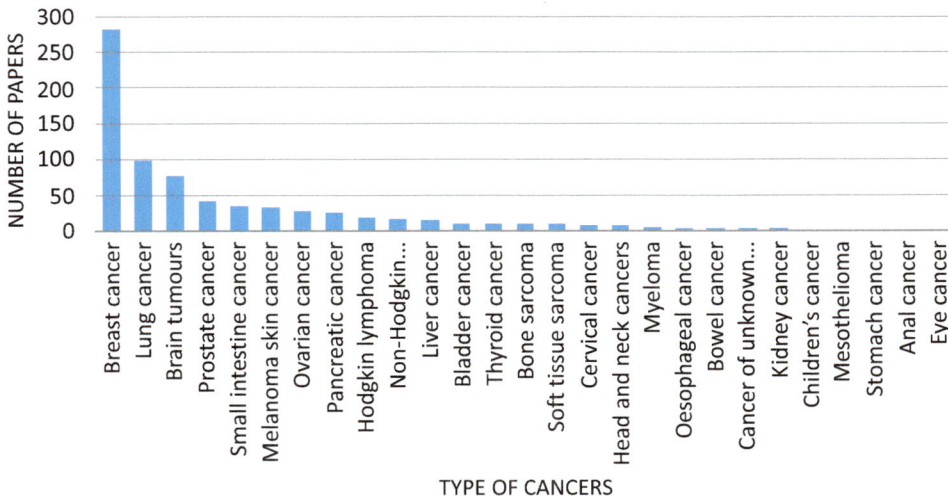

Fig. (2). Statistics of research literature on the application of AI technology in cancer diagnosis and treatment in the past decade.

3.2.2. Clinical Decision Support: Intelligent Data Integration

The development of four sub-fields of AI (machine learning, artificial neural networks, natural language processing, computer vision) has created favorable conditions for the development of the surgical field, mainly reflected in big data analysis, the establishment of intelligent shared databases, and the provision of favorable clinical decision support [28]. At present, the application of AI in surgical operations is in the stage of exploration and conception. In the future, surgeons will use intelligent analysis to obtain specific data for each stage of the patient's operation: before the operation, the mobile application and body tracker will automatically measure the weight, blood sugar, nutrition, activity, and other data of the surgical patient and provide electronic feedback based on the medical records, and automatic analysis of preoperative clinical data, to provide doctors with a more specific risk assessment of the surgical plan so that the prognosis of the surgery leads to a valuable prediction. During the operation, the mobile smart device integrates real-time analysis data of the surgical process, such as surgical video, vital signs, instrument monitoring results, high-frequency electrocautery energy use, *etc.* The surgeon can make the surgical process based on the integrated analysis results more accurate in terms of surgical, clinical decision-making and reduce or avoid the occurrence of adverse events. After the operation, the smart device will perform an integrated analysis of all the data before, during, and after the operation to help the patient understand the postoperative recovery status and effectively predict the complications. After discharge, the body tracker will continue to record the data after the patient is discharged, and analyze and integrate this data with the data of the perioperative period since the patient was admitted, and truly implement the patient-centered surgical nursing practice [29]. In addition, the smart device aggregates and uploads the video data collected during the operation (especially the captured surgical video of rare cases) to a shared intelligent database to promote the exchange of technology-based surgical practices, thereby improving the global surgical practice level [30 - 31]. Although intelligent data integration currently requires a combination of computer technical support and professional surgical practice, with the opening of the intelligent field of surgery, it will be realized in the near future in order to provide a basis for surgeons to make decisions [32]. It provides support and improves the accuracy of clinical, surgical decision-making.

4. THINKING AND PROSPECT

Although the development of AI has made great progress, compared with the development of AI itself, the application of AI in the medical field is still relatively lagging, and there is a lot of room for development and application [33 -

38]. It requires researchers to continue to broaden their horizons, use systematic and professional methods to explore the feasible path of the problem, deal with the current bottleneck of combining AI and medicine, and apply AI to the medical field in a targeted manner, and maximize the potential of AI and medicine. But there are also two points worth noting: One is the interpretability of the results of AI applications. As mentioned before, AI technology can reach a high level on the negative side of diagnostic accuracy, but the possibilities for obtaining excellent results are different in the "black box" state; therefore, strengthening the interpretability of AI technology in the medical field is still an important issue. The second is privacy and data security assurance; how to safely save data and comply with medical ethics is a problem that cannot be ignored in the development of AI. Every day, the hospital generates a large amount of complicated data, including patient information, medical records, medical imaging, pathology, laboratory examinations, and clinical diagnosis and treatment information. The availability of data is bound to affect patient privacy; the risk of data leakage will cause unimaginable losses. Therefore, further changes and development of AI in medicine are worth looking forward to.

CONSENT FOR PUBLICATION

Not Applicable.

CONFLICT OF INTEREST

The author confirms that this chapter contents have no conflict of interest.

ACKNOWLEDGEMENT

Declared none.

REFERENCES

[1]   Obermeyer Z, Emanuel EJ. Predicting the future - big data, machine learning,and clinical medicine. N Engl J Med 2016; 375(13): 1216-9.
        [http://dx.doi.org/10.1056/NEJMp1606181] [PMID: 27682033]

[2]   Bellman R. An introduction to artificial intelligence: can computer think?. San Francisco: Boyd & Fraser Pub Co. 1978; p. 1.

[3]   Yang J, Fong S, Li T. Attribute Reduction Based on Multi-objective Decomposition-Ensemble Optimizer with Rough Set and Entropy. 2019 International Conference on Data Mining Workshops (ICDMW). 673-80.
        [http://dx.doi.org/10.1109/ICDMW.2019.00102]

[4]   Hu Q, Yang J, Qin P, *et al.* Could or could not of Grid-Loc: grid BLE structure for indoor localisation system using machine learning. SOCA 2020.

[5]   Yang J, Ji Z, Liu S, *et al.* Multi-objective optimization based on pareto optimum in secondary cooling and EMS of continuous casting[C]//2016 International Conference on Advanced Robotics and Mechatronics (ICARM). IEEE. 283-7.

[6]   Jamshidi MB, *et al.* Artificial intelligence and COVID-19: deep learning approaches for diagnosis and treatment. IEEE Access.
        [http://dx.doi.org/10.1109/ACCESS.2020.3001973]

[7]   Galatenko VV, Lebedev AE, Nechaev IN, Shkurnikov MY, Tonevitskii EA, Podol'skii VE. On the construction of medical test systems using greedy algorithm and support vector machine. Bull Exp Biol Med 2014; 156(5): 706-9.
        [http://dx.doi.org/10.1007/s10517-014-2430-3] [PMID: 24770763]

[8]   Chen JH, Asch SM. Machine learning and prediction in medicine—beyond the peak of inflated expectations. N Engl J Med 2017; 376(26): 2507-9.
        [http://dx.doi.org/10.1056/NEJMp1702071] [PMID: 28657867]

[9]   De Wang. TOP100 cases in artificial intelligence 2019. Internet Weekly 2020(08): 30-47.

[10]   https://www.un.org/zh/sections/issues-depth/ageing/index.html

[11]   Kajitani I, Wakita Y. An Introduction to the Development of Transfer Assistive Robots in Japan[C]//AAATE Conf. 465-71.

[12]   Sedenberg E, Chuang J, Mulligan D. Designing commercial therapeutic robots for privacy preserving systems and ethical research practices within the home. Int J Soc Robot 2016; 8(4): 575-87.
        [http://dx.doi.org/10.1007/s12369-016-0362-y]

[13]   Holanda LJ, Silva PMM, Amorim TC, Lacerda MO, Simão CR, Morya E. Robotic assisted gait as a tool for rehabilitation of individuals with spinal cord injury: a systematic review. J Neuroeng Rehabil 2017; 14(1): 126.
        [http://dx.doi.org/10.1186/s12984-017-0338-7] [PMID: 29202845]

[14]   https://zh.unesco.org/themes/ethics-science-and-technology/comest

[15]   Liu Huang. Artificial intelligence AI has landed in various medical institutions in Britain and the United States. President of the Chinese Hospital 2017(12): 82-3.

[16]   Hogarty DT, Mackey DA, Hewitt AW. Current state and future prospects of artificial intelligence in ophthalmology: a review. Clin Exp Ophthalmol 2019; 47(1): 128-39.
        [http://dx.doi.org/10.1111/ceo.13381] [PMID: 30155978]

[17]   Suzuki K. Overview of deep learning in medical imaging. Radiological Phys Technol 2017; 10(3): 257-73.
        [http://dx.doi.org/10.1007/s12194-017-0406-5] [PMID: 28689314]

[18]   Di Cataldo S, Ficarra E. Mining textural knowledge in biological images: Applications, methods and trends. Comput Struct Biotechnol J 2016; 15: 56-67.
        [http://dx.doi.org/10.1016/j.csbj.2016.11.002] [PMID: 27994798]

[19]   Das DK, Chakraborty C, Bhattacharya PS. Automated screening methodology for asthma diagnosis that ensembles clinical and spirometric information. J Med Biol Eng 2016; 36(3): 420-9.
        [http://dx.doi.org/10.1007/s40846-016-0137-9]

[20]   Topalovic M, Laval S, Aerts JM, Troosters T, Decramer M, Janssens W. Automated interpretation of pulmonary function tests in adults with respiratory complaints. Respiration 2017; 93(3): 170-8.
        [http://dx.doi.org/10.1159/000454956] [PMID: 28088797]

[21]   Amaral JLM, Lopes AJ, Veiga J, Faria ACD, Melo PL. High-accuracy detection of airway obstruction in asthma using machine learning algorithms and forced oscillation measurements. Comput Methods Programs Biomed 2017; 144: 113-25.
        [http://dx.doi.org/10.1016/j.cmpb.2017.03.023] [PMID: 28494995]

[22]   Yao X, Abraham NS, Alexander GC, *et al.* Effect of adherence to oral anticoagulants on risk of stroke and major bleeding among patients with atrial fibrillation. J Am Heart Assoc 2016; 5(2)e003074
        [http://dx.doi.org/10.1161/JAHA.115.003074] [PMID: 26908412]

[23]   Zhou M, Chang HY, Segal JB, Alexander GC, Singh S. Adherence to a novel oral anticoagulant among patients with atrial fibrillation. J Manag Care Spec Pharm 2015; 21(11): 1054-62.
[http://dx.doi.org/10.18553/jmcp.2015.21.11.1054] [PMID: 26521117]

[24]   Huang S, Yang J, Fong S, Zhao Q. Artificial intelligence in cancer diagnosis and prognosis: Opportunities and challenges. Cancer Lett 2020; 471: 61-71.
[http://dx.doi.org/10.1016/j.canlet.2019.12.007] [PMID: 31830558]

[25]   Siegel RL, Miller KD, Jemal A. Cancer statistics, 2019. CA Cancer J Clin 2019; 69(1): 7-34.
[http://dx.doi.org/10.3322/caac.21551] [PMID: 30620402]

[26]   Papachristou Nikolaos, Puschmann Daniel, Barnaghi Payam, *et al.* Learning from data to predict future symptoms of oncology patients. PLOS ONE (2018)13(12): e0208808.
[http://dx.doi.org/10.1371/journal.pone.0208808]

[27]   Kamdar M, Centi A J, Agboola S, *et al.* A randomized controlled trial of a novel artificial intelligence-based smartphone application to optimize the management of cancer-related pain. J Clinical Oncology 2019; 36(34): 76.

[28]   Huang S, Yang J, Fong S, Zhao Q. Mining prognosis index of brain metastases using artificial intelligence. Cancers (Basel) 2019; 11(8): 1140.
[http://dx.doi.org/10.3390/cancers11081140] [PMID: 31395825]

[29]   Chen JH, Asch SM. Machine learning and prediction in medicine—beyond the peak of inflated expectations. N Engl J Med 2017; 376(26): 2507-9.
[http://dx.doi.org/10.1056/NEJMp1702071] [PMID: 28657867]

[30]   Kenngott HG, Wagner M, Nickel F, *et al.* Computer-assisted abdominal surgery: new technologies. Langenbecks Arch Surg 2015; 400(3): 273-81.
[http://dx.doi.org/10.1007/s00423-015-1289-8] [PMID: 25701196]

[31]   Volkov M, Hashimoto DA, Rosman G, *et al.* Machine learning and coresets for automated real-time video segmentation of laparoscopic and robot-assisted surgery[C]//2017 IEEE International Conference on Robotics and Automation (ICRA). IEEE. 754-9.

[32]   Yang J, Huang SG, Tang R. Broad Learning with Attribute Selection for Rheumatoid Arthritis, in: IEEE International Conference on Systems, Man and Cybernetics (SMC), IEEE, Toronto 2020.

[33]   Hu Q, Yang J, Qin P, Fong S. Towards a Context-Free Machine Universal Grammar (CF-MUG) in Natural Language Processing. IEEE Access 2020; 8: 165111-29.
[http://dx.doi.org/10.1109/ACCESS.2020.3022674]

[34]   Yang J, Ji Z, Liu S, Jia Q. Multi-objective optimization based on pareto optimum in secondary cooling and EMS of continuous casting. International Conference on Advanced Robotics and Mechatronics (ICARM). 283-7.
[http://dx.doi.org/10.1109/ICARM.2016.7606933]

[35]   Hu Q, Yang J, Qin P, Fong S, Guo J. Could or could not of Grid-Loc: grid BLE structure for indoor localisation system using machine learning. Serv Oriented Comput Appl 2020.
[http://dx.doi.org/10.1007/s11761-020-00292-z]

[36]   Yang J, Fong S, Li T. Attribute Reduction Based on Multi-objective Decomposition-Ensemble Optimizer with Rough Set and Entropy[C]//2019 International Conference on Data Mining Workshops (ICDMW). IEEE 2021; 673-80.

[37]   Hu Q, Yang J, Qin P, Fong S, Guo J. Could or could not of Grid-Loc: grid BLE structure for indoor localisation system using machine learning. Serv Oriented Comput Appl 2020.
[http://dx.doi.org/10.1007/s11761-020-00292-z]

[38]   Peng M, Yang J, Shi Q, *et al.* Artificial Intelligence Application in COVID-19 Diagnosis and Prediction 2020.

CHAPTER 3

Rethinking Artificial Intelligence in China's COVID-19 Pandemic

Qichao Wang[1,*]

¹ School of International Relations, Xi'an International Studies University, Xi'an, China

Abstract: The COVID-19 outbreak is currently rampant worldwide. The situation in China has been the toughest since the very beginning of the outbreak. However, the pace of the spread has been controlled after employing various policies to eliminate the further painful loss. The advancement of high technology in AI, big data, and machine learning has benefited mankind significantly, especially in this global public health crisis. This paper aims to rethink China's experiences in the application of AI from the concept of the "general-purpose technology" and attempts to link the technical aspect of AI to the future of Chinese society and culture regarding this technology.

Keywords: Artificial Intelligence, China, COVID-19, General-purpose technology.

1. INTRODUCTION

Artificial intelligence (AI) is a strategic technology leading the current technological revolution, industrial transformation, and competition. Technical advancements in statistics and computer software have enabled computer engineers and health scientists to collaborate and improve prognosis [1]. The COVID-19 epidemic is both a challenge and an opportunity for the development of the AI industry. In general, the opportunities outweigh the challenges. AI is valuable in many fields such as education, healthcare, engineering, and integrated social governance [2]. Similarly, AI is widely applied in the prevention, control, and diagnosis of COVID-19. Artificial intelligence can also provide social assistance for the prevention and treatment of COVID-19 in emerging industries such as intelligent auxiliary diagnosis, telemedicine with the Internet of things, psychological rehabilitation, and service robotics. Even robots have been effectively utilized in the fight against the COVID-19 epidemic.

* **Corresponding author Qichao Wang:** School of International Relations, Xi'an International Studies University, Xi'an, China; Tel: 8615363586080, Fax: 8615363586080; E-mail: wqc0410@gmail.com

Shigao Huang and Jie Yang (Eds.)

2. THE COVID-19 AND AI APPLICATION IN CHINA

In January 2020, new coronavirus-infected pneumonia (later termed COVID-19 by World Health Organization) epidemic spread from Wuhan, the central province of China, to other areas. It is now found in almost every corner worldwide. In attempting to manage the pandemic, many national and local governments have introduced public policy interventions such as social distancing and the quarantining of individuals showing symptoms of COVID-19 [3].

On January 23, 2020, the Wuhan government announced a "lockdown" to curb the spread of the virus. The COVID-19 pandemic is a huge challenge and a test for China's emergency and public health management systems. The pandemic directly impacted normal life negatively, resulting in the suspension of several businesses for months. Therefore, controlling the spread of the virus and returning to normal life is urgent. A focus on economic growth and the "elimination of poverty" is supposed to be a priority for the Beijing government. During the disease outbreak, China banned international travel, enhanced the test capacity of the nucleic acid, and developed a public policy to ensure home isolation. China also shared its data to study the trend of virus development. Some other sophisticated approaches have used the latent features of auto-encoders to predict infection rates and identify similar groups of regions or countries by using big data. For example, Hu *et al*. [4] compiled a data set of accumulated and new confirmed cases in 31 provinces and cities of China.

The uncertainty and complexity of the virus emerged as a threat to the lives and health of citizens in multiple nations and significantly challenged the efficiency and governance of the central authorities. The advancement of high technology, such as Artificial Intelligence (AI) and big data, assisted the governments in controlling the infectious disease during the struggle. China was considered the first country to mass-report cases of infection from numerous hospitals in patients and medical workers in Wuhan. The knowledge and experience from the previous outbreak and response to Severe Acute Respiratory Syndrome (SARS) aided the Chinese government in dealing with the spread of the virus.

Having access to the relevant information to trace the travelling history of the population is crucial for control of the coronavirus. In modern societies, the formation of information resources significantly depends on big data regarding the information of the movement of the population, providing important technical support for the tracing of the targeted cases [5]. Big data is the sum of structured, semi-structured, or unstructured data generated by fixed or mobile devices. Based on the Internet, big data, due to its accessibility and shareable characteristics, can be transformed into information by the government for decision-making by analyzing and processing it. The government obtained the relevant information and made decisions to warn the citizens on numerous applications in smartphones as well as reducing the losses which may have been caused by the aimless and wasteful restriction.

2.1. Big Data, Population Management, and Transportation

The objects of the big data analysis system include hospitals, disease control centers, government agencies, enterprises, communities, and citizens. In the early stage of the COVID-19 outbreak, the roads were cut off in many places to prevent free movement of the people, and hence, the spread of the virus, which resulted in inconvenience in the daily life of people [6]. Some local governments have employed technology-based management approaches. For example, on February 11, 2020, in Hangzhou, which is one of the leading cities on digital governance in China, the existing data management platform (Alipay) was used, which required the citizens to apply for health QR codes through the data platform [7]. Similarly, the Shenzhen-based technological company Tencent also developed relevant functions in its widely installed app, "WeChat." Big data provides the travelling history of the citizens and monitors their health status by a division of "green codes," "yellow codes," and "red codes," indicating the severity and relevance to the COVID-19 virus. The green code on the phone display allows the citizens to travel freely, while the yellow code and red code indicate that someone does not currently meet the satisfactory standard. The person would need to be monitored according to the regulation until the green code is achieved. In the age of big data, massive amounts of data are generated in real life. The search, analysis, and use of big data play an important role in public health emergency management and decision-making.

One of the important features confirming the presence of COVID-19 infection in patients is the body temperature. Therefore, monitoring the temperature of the mobile population, especially in densely populated areas (train stations, airports, subways, *etc.*), is essential for timely detection of the infection. It would help prevent the spread of the pandemic [8]. Traditional manual security check requires physical contact, leading to the risk of cross. A temperature measurement system based on image recognition technology and infrared thermal imaging technology can detect the human body and locate the target, thus can quickly identify and screen abnormal body temperature. To fulfill early warning by using pedestrian positioning, tracking and face recognition technology, one can also cooperate with high-risk personnel to perform isolation tasks. The automatic temperature monitoring products launched by Chinese domestic companies such as Baidu, Shangtang, Kuanggai, Dahua, Hikvision, *etc.*, have been widely used in public places such as train stations, airports, subway stations, and communities. They can detect multiple people in real-time at the same time with an identification error ± 0.3°C. Since there is no contact during the whole process, the efficiency is greatly improved.

The application of big data regarding the COVID-19 has improved the efficiency of government emergency management, and the color-based QR code as applied in China is the easiest way to make sense and operational among the citizens. The government can infer the probability and chronicles of public health events based on the data information generated to trace the travelling and contact history of the various cases, thus improving the accuracy and predictability of government decisions, warning the public in advance to avoid risks, and improving the government's capabilities in response to emergencies. The shared data can reduce the information asymmetry between the government and the public, and improve the credibility of the government. The collection of public health-related data indeed required a vast workload and a long-term data analysis, which poses a greater challenge to be more cooperation between the decision-making institutions and the professionals.

At present, the governments have built information platforms, and the big data information plays different roles for preemption, emergency management, and recovery in a post-epidemic era. Under the environment of big data sharing, the on-site data of emergencies are searched and quickly transmitted to various local governments, especially authorities dealing with the public contingency. The public also allows getting the updates and stimulating their willingness as citizens to involve in the control of the COVID-19 pandemic. Private enterprises, particularly the high-tech-driven companies involving in AI-based research and development, will reduce casualties and economic losses.

2.2. AI-based Medical System Against COVID in China

China has a vast territory and a large population, and there are certain gaps in the allocation of medical resources between different regions. Compared with medical staff and equipment, AI systems can be rapidly deployed through the big data storing in the cloud to prevent and control epidemic situations in underdeveloped areas and the grassroots units, to some extent alleviate the imbalanced medical resources [9].

The application of AI also assisted in reducing the risk of infection and ensure the safety of medical and healthcare workers. The Computed Tomography (CT) instrument equipped with an AI-assisted system can accurately recognize the position information of the face and the whole body without removing the mask.

In the whole process, the medical workers do not need to enter the scanning room, thereby significantly reducing the risk of cross-infection. Meanwhile, AI systems can improve the accuracy of checks. Besides, AI can also be associated with diagnosing contact history, clinical and laboratory data, biochemical indicators, nucleic acid test results, *etc.*, to further improve the accuracy of COVID-19 related medical checks [10].

2.3. AI-Based Public Policy Against COVID-19 in China

On March 24, the China AI Industry Alliance launched the report on AI and the Prevention and Control of the COIVD-19, in which the AI-based applications highly spoke for epidemic prevention and control, such as service robots, big data analysis systems, and intelligent identification (real-time temperature, facial recognition) products are the most used AI products in epidemic prevention and control.

The report sorted out more than 500 AI anti-epidemic cases collected by the "Artificial Intelligence Supporting New Coronary Pneumonia Epidemic Prevention and Control Information Platform", and summarized that the application of AI in this epidemic prevention and control covered six aspects, like epidemic monitoring and analysis, personnel management, Material provision, logistics support, drug research and development, medical treatment, and resumption of production [6].

As the Chinese president Xi Jinping pointed out, "we should encourage the use of digital technologies such as big data, AI, cloud computing, *etc.* to play a supporting role in epidemic monitoring and analysis, virus tracing, prevention and treatment, resource allocation, *etc.*" [6]. The Ministry of Industry and Information Technology also issued a proposal on "Fully exploiting the power of AI to fight against the COVID-19". It proposed to further apply AI products and services to effectively support epidemic prevention and control. From far-infrared thermal imaging, non-contact rapid temperature measurement to auxiliary diagnosis technology, from intelligent epidemic tracking based on big data, contactless distribution of robots to a remote office, AI products and applications are prevalent everywhere.

2.4. AI Enterprises and Societal Research And Development in China

The outbreak coincided with the Chinese Spring Festival resulting in large mobility and social gathering with a higher risk of cross-infection. Especially the virus has a "window period" of about 2-3 weeks. Thus how to accurately check and track high-risk personnel afterward is a major challenge for epidemic prevention. Measurements such as data mining technology to quickly screen and analyze mobile phone roaming information, consumption record, and traffic travel data, *etc.*, to extract the information of population mobility. To fulfill this task, Baidu, Sogou, 360 and other Chinese companies have launched information service systems such as epidemic tracking apps, and co-vehicle history checks. Didi and other online car reservation platforms have introduced traceable passenger travel records, which greatly facilitate relevant stakeholders and ordinary users to self-examine the risk of the epidemic situation on time.

During the epidemic, work from home (WFH) by online software abruptly remained the mainstream working style until late April in China. Cloud computing, artificial intelligence, big data, mobile Internet and other related technologies are comprehensively used in online document share and remote video conferences. For example, Xunfei from the Hong Kong University of Science and Technology (HKUST) developed a smart education standard solution for the students' self-learning purpose besides the regular live broadcast teaching, which summarized the most appropriate learning approach according to the students' knowledge background. Besides, HKUST's latest C-end office product is also based on AI. The application in the office scenario has made a series of technological innovations such as real-time "video-audio" script transfer by AI algorithm. The cloud storage and voice search function embodies the advantages of the high efficiency and convenience of AI in written and voice records in working, studying and living settings. Baidu, the largest searching engine and a very productive technological enterprise in Mainland China developed its epidemic map providing real-time big data reports on the COVID-19 mapping, including epidemic distribution and dynamics, migration and real-time broadcast of the epidemic. The searchable tracing of the co-vehicle transportation service updates information in real-time based on disclosed data for the public to check whether there are confirmed cases of new pneumonia in public places such as airplanes, trains, and buses.

A large number of AI technologies have been put into practical application in the prevention and control of the epidemic, which fully demonstrates that the new generation of information technology featured by AI and big data has been increasingly commercialized on the demand of the market and popularized through the rapid development and practice accumulation in the early stage. It also indicated that the scale of China's AI industry and the digital economy continues to grow and develop, and the integration with the economy continues to deepen, the shape of the intelligent society gradually emerges as well as demonstrating a good momentum of vigorous development [11]. Since the transmission approach has been detected, the main task of AI-based application is to establish epidemiological modeling to forecast national and local statistics with three dimensions: the total number of confirmed cases, the mortal rate and the recovery rates. When China has fully controlled the domestic situation, the Beijing government partially focused on forecasting the global trends of the pandemic to make policies towards foreign nations. It is safe to say the AI-based forecast modeling will also be utilized in the recovery of the global tourism industry and commercial flight business, the two sectors with disastrous aftermath brought by the COVID-19.

3. AI AS A GENERAL-PURPOSE TECHNOLOGY OF COVID-19 IN CHINA

Wuhan is the center for the outbreak of COVID-19 in China, a city that possesses more than 10 million population. With the pandemic of the pathogens, China, the largest country in terms of population, has put on a serious governmental philosophy and approach of the AI in its society, where the "human enhancing innovations" (HEI) has been put on agendas to imply with AI as a general-purpose technology (GPT). The most important general-purpose technology of our era is AI, particularly machine learning, that is, the machine's ability to keep improving its performance without humans having to explain exactly how to accomplish all the tasks. Within just the past few years, machine learning has become far more effective and widely available. We can now build systems that learn how to perform tasks on their own [12]. In the first sector, the overall situation about the pandemic prevention and control by the AI-based approaches has been briefly analyzed. Mokyr [13] made the arguments from the historic experiences that AI will amply its benign potential as a powerful technological force, and have to be settled down in the quite concrete institutional background (the government policy, citizen cultures and sponsorship of the entrepreneurial companies), in light of the overall political-economic considerations that providing the soil of the new GPT era of AI in such a global challenging time.

The multidisciplinary nature of the AI-based systems in the context of COVID-19 calls for the creation of a hybrid of global research teams and partnerships. As a result, the global funding opportunities also facilitate international collaborations and re-shape the research priorities among international communities to accelerate the success of the partnerships.

As mentioned in Trajtenberg [14], the development of AI has brought about a wave of complementary innovations in a wide and ever-expanding range of applications sectors. He framed three layers to elaborate how the AI created the division of "winner" and "loser" in such sweeping transformative processes, the education, personal services and direction of technical change, which also corroborates the current trend of the Chinese technology community with the influence the COVID-19.

The first layer of the analysis system is the theme of education. AI-based technology has become the dominant GPT in China and impacting the growth of every industry, thus, the required large-scale financial input and the education of the skilled human resources and the striking "ed-tech" (education-related technology) are the key domains assuring the success of China's AI industry, highly associated with personal services and the technical direction. In recent years, China has rushed to pursue "intelligent education". Now billion-dollar ed-tech companies are planning to export their vision overseas [15]. The COVID-19 and the current "de-coupling" between China and the US making China realize the enhancement of the AI-relevant industry is the only way to shrug off the "stranglehold problems" and without doubt, the ed-tech is the crucial strategic approach to fulfill the national AI development plan, and to some extent, it is perceived as the first but firm step.

In July 2017, China published its national guidance for AI development plan [16], in which it emphasized that AI-based technology should be taken into account for the curriculum of various education circles from elementary school to higher education. This direction of technical change is reiterated in the 19th National Congress of the Communist Party of China (CCP) in the same year. As the new age of AI approaches, China is looking at a variety of new strategies and approaches in the field of education, with its sights on both the long-term and the immediate basis, in basic as well as higher education, laying out a comprehensive AI strategy for a skilled workforce and civic education. The country also has a large number of hi-tech enterprises actively participating in exploring how the use of AI can change education [17]. Besides, the "study from home" (SFH) in the COVID-19 utilized the distance education approach to keep the students at all levels in mind that the AI-based distance learning and studying is a "turnover" experience comparing to the in-class learning activity. The multiple apps installed in their smartphones or other devices drew a 360° "panorama" atmosphere to the "ed-tech" products, which subsequently encouraged the technical professionals to participate in the effort to popularize AI education and improve the nurture of the AI production among the developer, entrepreneur, and consumer. The usefulness of all types of platforms for AI innovation is fully realized in scientific education, museums and automatically steps into the second layer of the analysis system, the personal services.

In 2015, the US Bureau of Labor Statistics researched to forecast AI's impact on the development of the personal service to the next ten years as Table **1**:

Table 1. US employment by major sector.

	Millions			**Percentage Growth***
Sector	2014	2024*	Change*	-
Goods-producing	19	19	-	+7%
Services	121	130	+9.3	+20%
Of which: healthcare & social assistance	18	22	+3.8	+1
Other	10	11	+0.5	+6%
Total	151	160	+9.8	

Source: Occupational employment projections to 2024, Monthly Labor Review, U.S. Bureau of Labor Statistics, December 2015. https://www.bls.gov/opub/mlr/2015/article/occupational-employment-projectios-to-2024.htm

The research took the change in the nursery professionals in the US after the second world war to demonstrate how a correlational upgrading is taking place in the advancement of the nursery profession including salary, educational level, and technologies that benefitted from the technological advancements as highlighted in the above survey, the occupations such as health care and social assistance (nurses, caregiving) will be a great beneficiary from the advent of AI, which smartly interfaces between the practitioners of these occupations and the AI-based machine learning.

The survey not only predicts the US's AI-related personal services but also precisely forecasts what is happening in China due to the rise of the middle class and the continuous technological-based economy.

The application of big data and AI in the medical field has also promoted changes in medical service models and health management concepts. Nowadays, people do not necessarily need to go to the hospital to run daily health management. Through smart wearable devices and home intelligent health detection and monitoring equipment, which can dynamically monitor health data in real-time and accurately grasp personal health conditions.

In China, the vigorous development of AI has promoted the progress of basic medical research, opened up a broad space for precision medicine, and strengthened the confidence of humans in defeating various diseases, which is perceived as one of the most important personal services that Chinese most-often used. The COVID-19 pandemic reinforced the habits of the application of big data and AI-based apps to warn, forecast, and detect the possible and suspect situation and triggered a more popular culture of the utilization of AI-based solutions among Chinese citizens. For example, as the prevalence of Alipay, Wechat and the AI-based wearing products (Xiaomi, Huawei) and apps, Chinese people are now willing to utilize these personal services to examine their health status and form a routine of daily exercises. The Wechat can calculate how many steps you forwarded in a day and make a competition with your other Wechat friends, which makes it easier to keep people doing various health-related sports. Moreover, due to the involvement of AI in the health industry, small checks, such as blood pressure, heart rate, can be conducted by the AI-based product used at home with less or no visiting hospital or doctor consultation, giving the medical workers more space to solve sophisticated problems and diseases using AI auxiliary approaches. AI can provide normalized and refined guidance to provide comprehensive and full-cycle health services for specific groups. These are not only conducive to strengthening disease prevention and improving the efficiency of chronic disease management, but also can enhance the public's health concept and fundamentally save the medical cost of the whole society.

The direction of the technical change as the third and last layer addressed the future relations between AI and human beings. As AI is the dominant GPT in the contemporary international community, there is a long-existing debate about the relationship between AI and mankind for the topics such as job market, the new skilled human resources with two different directions: the human enhancing innovation (HEI) and human replacing innovation (HRI). We label these "human-enhancing innovations" ("HEI"). Take the medical industry, for example, the AI doesn't replace doctors (partially but will never be full) but rather augment their human-bound capabilities (the medical robot surgery). AI-based HEI's have the potential to unleash a new wave of human creativity and productivity, particularly in services, whereas HRI's either decrease employment (*e.g.* Telsa) or create unworthy jobs [16]. However, the work from home (WFH) drew a great dilemma: the remote working pattern may incept a new relational work-life balance in the future: AI helped the companies achieve more tasks than that of the previous deployment of the human resources plan. The global economy due to the COVID-19 implied a more jobless market ahead of the employees, but AI replaced the smart machine with a man in many of the jobs, thus the "human-machine" crisis demonstrates its new trend during the pandemic.

4. CONCLUSION

The AI and machine learning against COVID-19 and post-pandemic global research are tremendously highlighted by a prospectus of international cooperation to maximize the potential of high technology. The breakthrough of the AI-based fight against COVID-19 including the vaccine is one of the achievements from the international cooperation and should be shared as a public good as China's President Xi Jinping proposed. From a societal perspective, AI has been applied in several areas of epidemiological research modeling empirical data, including forecasting the number of cases given in different public policy choices. With the continued growth of the COVID-19 pandemic, researchers worldwide are working to better understand, mitigate, and suppress its spread. Key areas of research include studying COVID-19 transmission, facilitating its testing process, developing possible vaccines and treatments, and understanding the socio-economic impacts of the pandemic [18].

Many recent publications in some leading medical journals such as Nature, JAMA revealed the contribution from AI regarding the molecular drug, the individual patient diagnosis, but still, very limited research is conducted to its use on a societal scale. Some social sciences of info-demic, social trust and equality discussion and "handbook" for the citizens living in a "post-COVID-19" society is also needed. Social media and other online data sources can also provide a rich source of information for understanding public opinion, perception and behaviour. For example, Liu *et al* [19] combined related internet search and news media activity with data from the Chinese Center for Disease Control and daily forecasts from GLEAM [20], an agent-based mechanistic model, to produce 2-day forecasts for a range of daily statistics. The authors first clustered provinces based on geo-spatial similarities in COVID-19 activity and then trained a separate model on each cluster.

The role of AI in various industries has become increasingly apparent. In the process of helping epidemic prevention and control, AI technology integrates with new-generation information technologies such as 5G, big data, blockchain, industrial Internet, Internet of Vehicles, *etc.* in accordance with the principle of "possible and necessary", stepping up upgrades and transformations, exploring innovation. Traditional products of various industries, a batch of new products and formats have emerged in large numbers, which has greatly expanded the new space of the AI industry in the future.

In the post-epidemic society, the full-scale resumption of production, and with the real-time implementation of the "new infrastructure", AI will further integrate with manufacturing, transportation, agriculture and other basic industries to promote the intelligent upgrade of the industry. AI is of great significance for furthering the development of the technical and economic world [21]. Moreover, AI and other technologies can play vital roles in enhancing national governance capabilities and gradually becoming more prominent. The epidemic fully demonstrated the advantages of AI technology in solving national governance problems and improving the modernization of national comprehensive governance capabilities. For example, the application of AI in epidemic monitoring, risk analysis and early warning, and transportation travel is essential to enhance the capabilities of smart cities and governance [22 - 24]. Through powerful big data collection and intelligent analysis, combined with social governance theory and high technology, the complex social operation system is mapped into a multi-dimensional, dynamic data system [25], realizing real-time, quantitative and visual monitoring of social operation laws, and social preference. An early warning has effectively served the government's decision-making, guaranteed the people's right to know information, and ensured a good social order. It is foreseeable that in the future, with the continuous accumulation of social operating data features, AI will enter economic and political decision-making, control systems, and simulation systems to promote the transformation of traditional social governance into smart social governance. AI has become an important driving force for social and economic development.

CONSENT FOR PUBLICATION

Not Applicable.

CONFLICT OF INTEREST

The author confirms that this chapter contents have no conflict of interest.

ACKNOWLEDGEMENT

Declared none.

REFERENCES

[1]   Huang S, Yang J, Fong S, Zhao Q. Artificial intelligence in cancer diagnosis and prognosis: Opportunities and challenges. Cancer Lett 2020; 471: 61-71.
        [http://dx.doi.org/10.1016/j.canlet.2019.12.007] [PMID: 31830558]

[2]   Peng M, Yang J, Shi Q, *et al.* Artificial intelligence application in COVID-19 diagnosis and prediction. SSRN Electronic J 2020. https://ssrn.com/abstract=3541119

[3]   Yang Zifeng, Zeng Zhiqi, *et al.* SEIR and AI prediction of the trend of the epidemic of COVID-19 in China under public health interventions. J Thoracic Dis 2020; 12(3): 165-74.

[4]   Hu Z, Ge Q, Li S, Jin L, Xiong M. Artificial Intelligence Forecasting of COVID-19 in China. arXiv preprint arXiv:200207112 2020.

[5]   Ting DSW, Carin L, Dzau V, Wong TY. Digital technology and COVID-19. Nat Med 2020; 26(4): 459-61.
        [http://dx.doi.org/10.1038/s41591-020-0824-5] [PMID: 32284618]

[6]   Yu H, Sun X, Solvang WD, Zhao X. Reverse logistics network design for effective management of medical waste in epidemic outbreaks: Insights from the coronavirus disease 2019 (COVID-19) outbreak in Wuhan (China). Int J Environ Res Public Health 2020; 17(5): 1770.
        [http://dx.doi.org/10.3390/ijerph17051770] [PMID: 32182811]

[7]   Artificial Intelligence Industry Alliance Report. 2020. The e-version is available at http://pdf.dfcfw.com/pdf/H3_AP202003301377165861_1.pdf

[8]   Liu XX, Fong S. Towards a realistic model for simulating spread of infectious COVID-19 disease.

Proceedings of 2020 the 4th International Conference on Big Data and Internet of Things. 2020; pp. 96-101.

[9]   Allam Z, Jones DS. On the coronavirus (COVID-19) outbreak and the smart city network: universal data sharing standards coupled with artificial intelligence (AI) to benefit urban health monitoring and management. Healthcare (Basel) 2020; 8(1): 46.
[http://dx.doi.org/10.3390/healthcare8010046] [PMID: 32120822]

[10]   Ai Tao, Yang Zhenlu, Hou Hongyan, *et al.* Correlation of Chest CT and RT-PCR Testing in Coronavirus Disease 2019 (COVID-19) in China: A Report of 1014 Cases. Radiology 2020.

[11]   Hua J, Shaw R. Corona virus (COVID-19) "infodemic" and emerging issues through a data lens: the case of China. Int J Environ Res Public Health 2020; 17: 2309.
[http://dx.doi.org/10.3390/ijerph17072309]

[12]   Erik Brynjolfsson and Andrew Mcafee. 2017.The business of artificial intelligence
https://hbr.org/cover-story/2017/07/the-business-of-artificial-intelligence

[13]   Mokyr J. The Past and the Future of Innovation: some lessons from Economic History.

[14]   Trajtenberg M. AI as the next GPT: a political-economy perspective. National Bureau of Economic Research Working Paper 24245.
[http://dx.doi.org/10.3386/w24245]

[15]   Hao K. China has started a grand experiment in AI education. It could reshape how the world learns. MIT Technology Review Available at: https://www.technologyreview.com/2019/08/ 02/131198/ china-squirrel-has-started-a-grand-experiment-in-ai-education-it-could-reshape -how-the/

[16]   The National Guideline of Artificial Intelligence Development. State Council of China 2017.
http://www.gov.cn/zhengce/content/2017-07/20/content_5211996.htm?from=timeline&isappinstalled=0

[17]   Yang X. Accelerated move for AI education in China. ECNU Review of Education 2019; 2(3): 347-52.
[http://dx.doi.org/10.1177/2096531119878590]

[18]   Bullock J, Luccioni A, Hoffmann K. Mapping the landscape of Artificial Intelligence applications against COVID-19, 2020.https://arxiv.org/pdf/2003.11336.pdf

[19]   Liu D, Clemente L, Poirier C, Ding X, Chinazzi M, David JT, *et al.* A machine learning methodology for real-time forecasting of the 2019-2020 COVID-19 outbreak using Internet searches, news alerts, and estimates from mechanistic models. arXiv preprint arXiv:200404019.

[20]   Balcan D, Gonçalves B, Hu H, Ramasco JJ, Colizza V, Vespignani A. Modeling the spatial spread of infectious diseases: the GLobal Epidemic and Mobility computational model. J Comput Sci 2010; 1(3): 132-45.
[http://dx.doi.org/10.1016/j.jocs.2010.07.002] [PMID: 21415939]

[21]   Huang S, Yang J, Fong S, Zhao Q. Mining prognosis index of brain metastases using artificial intelligence. Cancers (Basel) 2019; 11(8): 11.
[http://dx.doi.org/10.3390/cancers11081140] [PMID: 31395825]

[22]   Hu Q, Yang J, Qin P, Fong S. Towards a context-free machine universal grammar (CF-MUG) in natural language processing. IEEE Access 2020; 8: 165111-29.
[http //dx.doi.org/10.1109/ACCESS.2020.3022674]

[23]   Yang J, Huang SG, Tang R. Broad Learning with Attribute Selection for Rheumatoid Arthritis, in IEEE International Conference on Systems, Man and Cybernetics (SMC), IEEE, Toronto, 2020.

[24]   Hu Q, Yang J, Qin P, Fong S, Guo J. Could or could not of Grid-Loc: grid BLE structure for indoor localisation system using machine learning. Serv Oriented Comput Appl 2020; 14: 61-174.
[http //dx.doi.org/10.1007/s11761-020-00292-z]

[25]　Yang J, Fong S, Li T. Attribute reduction based on multi-objective decomposition-ensemble optimizer with rough set and entropy. International Conference on Data Mining Workshops (ICDMW). IEEE 2019; pp. 673-80.

CHAPTER 4

Artificial Intelligence System and its Application in Clinical Oncology

Shigao Huang[1,*], Jie Yang[2,3], Qun Song[2], Kexing Liu[2], Simon Fong[2,4] and Qi Zhao[1]

[1] *Institute of Translational Medicine, Faculty of Health Sciences, University of Macau 999078, Macau SAR, China*

[2] *Department of Computer and Information Science, University of Macau, Macau, China*

[3] *Chongqing Industry and Trade Polytechnic, Chongqing, China*

[4] *Zhuhai Institutes of Advanced Technology of the Chinese Academy of Sciences, China*

Abstract: The essence of the Artificial Intelligence (AI) decision system is that it helps us to make a better clinical plan and improve decision efficiency. Mature systems need data, core algorithms, and good interface support. Based on the cancer database of the Chinese Society of Clinical Oncology and the domestic core algorithm, we created the AI decision system with independent intellectual property rights using I ~ IV phases of clinical trials and research. To verify the accuracy of the system, we need assistance from doctors at different levels. The promotion of this system will further improve the standardized diagnosis and treatment of breast cancer and provide guidance for the establishment and application of other intelligent decision-making systems.

Keywords: Artificial Intelligence System, Clinical oncology, Clinical validation, I-IV phase clinical trial.

1. INTRODUCTION

Cancer has become one of the main causes of death in China [1, 2]. Standardized treatment is an important measure to improve the cure rate and ensure the prognosis of patients. However, considering the differences in regional development and the accessibility of diagnosis and treatment means [3], there are still great differences in the standardization of diagnosis and treatment in China.

[*] **Corresponding author Shigao Huang:** Institute of Translational Medicine, Faculty of Health Sciences, University of Macau 999078, Macau SAR, China; Tel: 853 88222953, Fax: 853 88222953; E-mail: huangshigao2010@aliyun.com.
[#] SH and JY have equal contribution.

Meanwhile, tumor therapy has been developing rapidly in recent years. For example, in 2018, the number of new drugs approved by the US Food and Drug Administration (FDA) broke the record of the number of new drugs approved in previous years, among which anti-tumor drugs accounted for 27% of all the drugs.

The proliferation of new drugs and newly approved indications has put pressure on clinicians. However, due to limited energy and learning abilities, it is difficult for clinicians to quickly grasp the differences between different tumors and the best treatment plan, thus reducing the therapeutic effect. In my previous study, we used machine learning to determine cancer progress and diagnosis [4]. The AI decision system, namely the clinical decision Support System (CDSS), is a kind of search engine used to filter the best results from the knowledge base, developed through the key information and feedback provided by the users. CDSS can help clinical workers reduce dependence on memory, reduce error rate, reduce response time, and help them make appropriate and safe decisions in clinical work, ensuring clinical safety and quality, thus improving therapeutic effect [5].

CDSS can also help clinicians optimize treatment plans by integrating different data and providing personalized advice based on differences in drug efficacy, product accessibility, adverse reactions, patients' economic status, and health insurance level. After more than 20 years of development, CDSS has played an important role in disease management, radiotherapy dose calculation, ECG reading, blood bank system, and other fields [6 - 8]. Watson tumor System (WFO) was one of the early tumor treatment decision systems developed to provide help to clinicians according to the literature, protocol, case list, and by learning from the treatment experiences, *etc* [9].

Using the WFO system, our center conducted the first clinical study of an intelligent system in the field of breast cancer [8]. By comparing the advantages and disadvantages of WFO schemes, we explored the help AI systems provide to doctors at different levels, which enabled us to understand the role of intelligent decision making in clinical practice, and also found the efficacy of the WFO system in our national conditions.

We realised that no mature, intelligent system was being applied in cancer treatment in China. Thus, we established the first AI decision system under the Chinese Society of Clinical Oncology (CSCO) by using databases, guidelines, and technologies. The purpose of this paper is to discuss the development, verification, and promotion of the CSCO AI system and provide guidance for CDSS development and application in China.

2. DEVELOPMENT OF AN AI SYSTEM

A CDSS developed by employing AI must provide an accurate medical decision according to the needs of the individual patients. This system can only be developed if we have a reliable database that will lead us to build a knowledge map. Only then a clinical decision can be obtained automatically by using a friendly communication interface. The clinicians can go through the simple operation steps, get more effective information, and provide optimized treatment decisions.

2.1. Establish a Knowledge Base

The knowledge base is the cornerstone of the CSCO AI system, including system learning, testing, and verification. All its needs are based on the knowledge base.

The richness and representativeness of the knowledge base directly affect the reliability of the system. The knowledge base of the CSCO AI system mainly comes from clinical data and evidence-based medical evidence. The former is mostly semi-structured or unstructured, while the latter is structured data. The main source of clinical data is the electronic medical record system. Although China has adopted the international disease code and surgical classification code [10], these two terms still cannot cover all the clinical information in medical records.

At the same time, there are differences in the data structure and standards of the information systems established by major hospitals across the country, and the storage methods are also different. Therefore, the establishment of standardized and unified standard data sets is an important step to break the "information island" barrier in the era of Big Data [11].

The purpose of this article is to describe structured reporting and the development of large databases for use in data mining in breast imaging. The clinical and medical data of structured design, at the same time, will be dispersed in the different clinical information system of different hospitals through data collecting data and integration steps, such as cleaning, and the using natural language for the main index, technology, structures, and patients of breast cancer.

Since the establishment of the CSCO BC database in 2015, it has collected more than 50,000 cases of breast cancer diagnosis and treatment in different regions spanning more than 40 years in China. Some of the first domestic studies have been recorded, showing the changes in breast cancer diagnosis and treatment in China. This is an important data source for us to build the knowledge base, and also provides a database for subsequent system validation and testing.

Knowledgebase of a data source in the medical literature is programmed according to a different stage of breast cancer patients with an intent to automatically retrieve relevant clinical research on individual patients in the literature (such as different TNM staging, molecular classification, past drug use, adverse reactions, *etc.*). It is based on the literature summary, by the panel of clinicians, finally set up different types of tumor diagnosis and treatment of the patients with the of knowledge map [11, 12].

2.2. Building Knowledge Map

After the completion of data collection, it is necessary to integrate the data through technical means, map the abstract data into graphic elements, and supplement it with human-computer interaction means to help users effectively perceive and analyze the data [13]. Knowledge spectrogram can capture and present the intricate relationship between domain concepts and connect the fragmented knowledge fragments in various information systems. It plays a very important role in knowledge retrieval, question and answer, knowledge recommendation, knowledge visualization, and other applications. It also provides an ideal technical means to solve the problem of "data island", which is conducive to the integration of knowledge resources and the improvement of knowledge serviceability [14].

By constructing a knowledge map, the CSCO AI system extracts entity-relationship and forms a knowledge network structure similar to human understanding. For complex professional medical knowledge, the expert guidance of classified structured, the formation of tumor diagnosis, and treatment of knowledge collection for textual data is required under the specification of medical standard terminology to carry on the text analysis, such as semantic annotations, correlation analysis, and for all the concepts on the tumor diagnosis and data collection.

Then the interaction between the data and clinical workers is completed through semantic analysis, reasoning, and auxiliary diagnosis and treatment system. During use, CSCO AI can also feedback and update the system based on the patient's clinical diagnosis and treatment data. CSCO guideline [14, 15] is a guideline written keeping in mind China's national conditions. According to patients of different stages and different categories of breast cancer, different treatment decisions are made in combination with China's reality and the latest evidence-based medicine. The CSCO AI system builds different knowledge graphs based on the scheme in the guide and locates knowledge graphs based on the key pieces of information when users search for relevant information.

3. MAN-MACHINE COMMUNICATION INTERFACE

The human-machine communication interface plays an important role in interaction, and a reasonable communication interface is conducive to the promotion and application of the system, to improve the rationality of treatment [13, 16]. AI in breast cancer diagnosis and treatment is focused on the timeline, age, TNM stage, patients with input molecular classification, and other important information. The system is first to screen patients' basic situation and then to identify the key information before treatment.

Once the doctors select the recommended specific plan, they can link to the knowledge map centered on the treatment plan, presenting entity relations such as clinical evidence, references, usage, and dosage of relevant drugs, drug name and side effects of CSCO BC guidelines, and also synchronously link to the views of domestic experts on diagnosis and treatment, to generate views exchange.

CSCO AI will also integrate medical insurance, clinical research, and other data to make it more consistent with the domestic reality, to ensure that users can obtain more information by pressing a button, and enhance the efficiency of clinical workers.

4. AI CLINICAL VALIDATION

For secure application and better promotion of CDSS, this AI system needs to be optimized through clinical validation and user feedback. Fig. (1) showed that the flow chart of using Houyi Collector to mine machine learning methods applied in tumor prognosis prediction. Then, we divided the verification of the CSCO AI system into four stages, which include: the identification of effective information stage, decision-making stage, decision verification stage, and lastly, marketing stage. The purposes of each stage or phase of the research are different, and the employed research methods are also different.

4.1. Phase I Clinical Research

Identifying the integrity of valid information: AI system developed by the technicians in CSCO under the guidance of experts in the field of breast cancer is an intelligent system. Due to differences in the background of various clinical cases, there are chances of making an error in the diagnosis. So Phase I clinical research is based on the test and study of the cases of different stages, clinical history and backgrounds and different decisions are made by the clinicians in those cases. Thus Phase I provides the key information needed to set the priority of the information on which the subsequent decision and the guidelines are based.

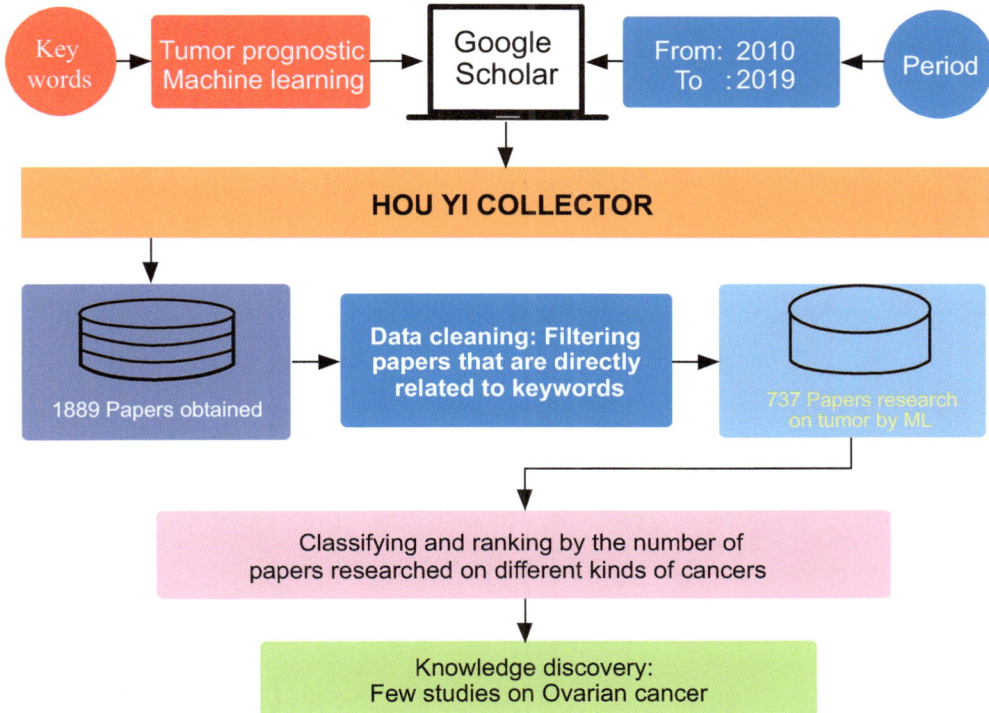

Fig. (1). The flow chart of using Houyi Collector in machine learning methods applied in tumor prognosis.

The first step in a research method is using the BC (breast cancer) data of the post-operation relapse, metastasis in patients with advanced breast cancer, screening for the initial treatment and postoperative adjuvant therapy for each patient. The probability of success of an intelligent decision-making system (AI), depends on the understanding and evaluating the key pieces of information provided in the database. Finally, the results of 200 patients with recurrent and metastatic breast cancer were screened from the CSCO BC database. Among them, 18% were triple-negative breast cancer (TNBC), 65% were hormone receptor-positive, and 32% were human epidermal growth factor receptor 2 (HER2) positive [17].

In the initial stage of treatment and postoperative adjuvant therapy, an intelligent decision scheme of the AI system is given, to satisfy the goals of Phase I clinical research. Thus, we explored that the AI system being prepared under CSCO can give reasonable treatment decisions in second-line therapy, laying a foundation for the application and expansion of the system. Although, the system still lacks a comprehensive understanding of some high-risk factors. For example, patients with a low histological grade but high KI67 are still treated as low-risk patients, and the wrong scheme is given. This part is modified by the developments in AI system in subsequent phases of clinical research.

4.2. Phase II Clinical Research

To investigate the efficacy of the clinical recommendation: After the completion of Phase I, the next step is verification *i.e.*, if the AI system developed can process the information given in the database, and the decision schemes developed under the AI system are applicable or not?. At this point, it remains to be seen whether the CSCO AI protocol conforms to the guidelines and whether it can be applied in the clinic.

Therefore, at the II phase of clinical research, a proposal is given to test its validation and accuracy or the extent of accuracy in different cases. It is also tested the decision system conforms to the guidelines of the Healthcare system or not [17]. We also evaluate if the decision system can be employed for the general public not. All these assessments lay the foundation for a decision system in the research, and its subsequent extension to III phase.

The random screening of recurrence metastasis from BC database, the first-line treatment of patients with breast cancer, analysis of the AI in the initial treatment, adjuvant therapy, first-line treatment, secondary treatment stage, decision-making, validation step AI decisions at different stages and testing the conformity degree of decision system are the steps involved in research methodology (got the AI plan and guidelines for Phase I ~ II and the recommended level of conformity degree).

To evaluate the results from the CSCO BC database, 300 patients were screened and 1200 tests were completed. The results showed that the decision scheme given by the CSCO AI system at different stages was different from the CSCO BC guidelines.

In neoadjuvant therapy, adjuvant radiotherapy, and adjuvant targeted therapy, the coincidence rate can reach 100% due to the clear indications and treatment plan.

However, the coincidence rate of adjuvant chemotherapy was only 88.2% [18], because the system could not give the decision recommendation in adjuvant therapy before neoadjuvant chemotherapy was completed. However, the follow-up treatment of patients with non-standard neoadjuvant therapy could not be clearly defined in clinical practice, so we modified the logic algorithm and did not recommend follow-up treatment for these patients.

For example, in patients with lymph node metastasis, if the patient does not have the KI67 index, the treatment recommendation cannot be given, which is inconsistent with the reality, and we have corrected this part. In the stage of recurrence and metastasis, due to the complexity of previous treatment, it is difficult to determine whether the drug is resistant or the drug can be reused, so the compliance rate with the guidelines is only 94.6% and 87.4% [19]. In clinical work, there is still a lack of a reliable standard for drug resistance, and there will be significant errors in the judgment of drug resistance. Therefore, we add the option of drug resistance and let clinical workers determine drug resistance to avoid ethical problems caused by systematic judgment errors. In Phase II clinical research notes, the AI system is verified with notes and BC guidelines. Resultantly, the overall coincidence rate can reach more than 95%, conforms with the clinical demand. We may also keep on improving the AI algorithms and mature the system further.

4.3. Phase III Clinical Research

In III phase clinical trial, we generally evaluate the survival of patients using the traditional statistic. Now, we may adopt machine learning to analyze the result and evaluate the III phase clinical research (Fig. **2**) and decision-making. III Phase clinical research is mainly based on randomized trials, exploring the extent to which AI systems can provide clinical help practically, thus further optimizing the interface at the same time, to facilitate its subsequent promotion.

Whether CDSS can optimize clinical decision-making, and how to evaluate the degree of optimization, are the some of questions to be answered in this phase. Although it is more meaningful to compare the acceptance of intelligent decisions by making plans or by conducting follow-up studies, there are still ethical bottlenecks, so the use of retrospective data is a common way to explore decision optimization [17].

Comparison of compliance rates between different protocols with the CSCO BC guidelines [20] or the National Comprehensive Cancer Network (NCCN) guidelines can assist in determining the differences between these groups [21]. Therefore, according to the two guidelines, we developed an evaluation scale for the verification of intelligent systems.

Decision-making plan if complying with the guidelines recommended high-level NCCN guidelines 1 kind of evidence or notes BC instructions I level and in line with the clinical practice [22], it is completely accord with, can be three points; If meet high level recommended but is not in conformity with the clinical practice, or conform to the NCCN guidelines 2 class a piece of evidence or notes BC instructions II level and in line with the clinical practice, for the high level, can be to 2 points; If do not conform to the guidelines, but in clinical practice, or conform to the NCCN guidelines only 2 b kind of evidence or notes BC guidelines recommended minimum to 1 III level; Failure to comply with guidelines and clinical practice will result in a score of 0. To ensure the relative rationality of the score, two experts with more than 10 years of clinical experience in the treatment of breast cancer were selected for independent scoring, and experts with more than 30 years of clinical experience of treatment of breast cancer with inconsistent scores were arbitrated to form the final score.

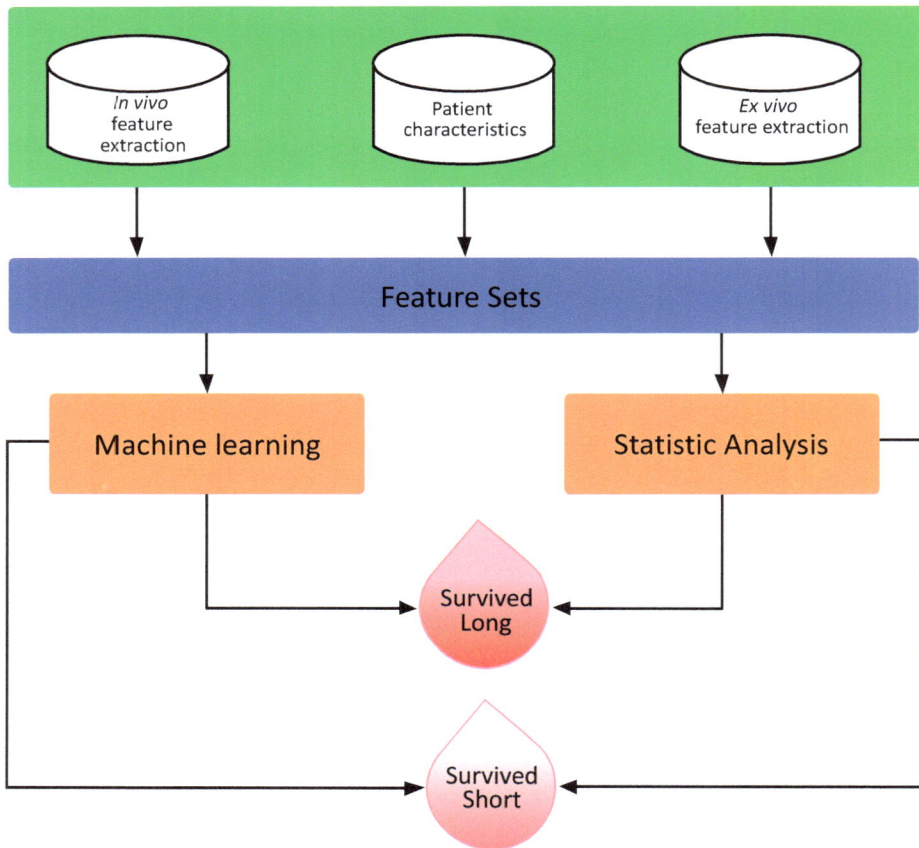

Fig. (2). The framework of ovarian cancer prognosis (machine learning *vs* traditional methods).

Clinical research design is the design created by different clinical researchers in the center by the WFO system [23]. The results showed that after reference WFO physician decision scheme with the original consistency of 56%, the consistency of different level doctor, significantly higher than that of chief physician and surgeon resident (68% and 54%;49%;P = 0.001).

It indicates that different doctors have different acceptance of the WFO system. We also used the decision evaluation scale to evaluate whether the protocol was more consistent with the guidelines after the change and to explore the practical significance of WFO for clinicians. We verified it through an Evaluation system to know the level of difference, by putting some clinicians to test.

Breast cancer cases at different stages and in different categories were screened from the CSCO BC database. After sorting out the questions, clinicians at different levels and backgrounds were screened. They were put to test and were asked to answer the questions according to the CSCO BC guidelines [20]. The intelligent decision Evaluation Scale (Table **1**) was used to check the score of doctors' who answered the questions, to compare the degree of compliance between the CSCO AI plan and doctors at different levels, and to determine with which level of doctors the CSCO AI plan is more consistent with. The results are being further analyzed.

Table 1. Intelligent Decision Evaluation Scale.

Grade	Score Requirement	Score
Exact match	Conform to NCCN I evidence and clinical practice	2
Intermediate match	Conform either NCCN I evidence or clinical practice	1
Not match	Not conform to both NCCN I evidence and clinical practice	0

4.4. Phase IV Clinical Research

Reliable Application with Safety and Effectiveness: After the completion of phase I ~ III study, we need AI systems to meet clinical needs, and can start marketing, popularization and application.

Phase IV clinical research involves the wide application of an AI system to investigate its reliability, optimizing the interface at the same time [24], and further expanding the application. Currently, intelligent doctor training has been conducted to help clinical workers better familiarize themselves with the CSCO AI system, and subsequently, it will be promoted and tested in designated hospitals nationwide. By collecting information through subsequent treatments, to understand the acceptance of AI system by different expters [25] according to their clinical needs, healthcare norms, economic factors, safety data, we came to know that now and then a new model is being proposed, such as bone marrow protection, liver damage prediction model, *etc* were developed, thus improving the scope of AI system, and resultantly promote intelligent management concept [26].

CSCO AI system is an intelligent decision system based on the Chinese core algorithm, CSCO BC guidelines, and database. So far, its application has been carried out in more than 30 hospitals. In the future, we will continue to optimize the CSCO AI system to make it more intelligent and make efforts to respond to the call of the "2030 Megaproject" - New Generation Artificial Intelligence.

Like clinical medicine, AI has its application in other fields such as engineering, natural language processing, bioinformatics, *etc* [27 - 31]. With a special focus on clinical diagnosis, as well as interpretability, AI is likely to remain an important issue in the future, and we are going to witness a widespread use of AI technology and its applications.

CONSENT FOR PUBLICATION

Not Applicable.

CONFLICT OF INTEREST

The author confirms that this chapter contents have no conflict of interest.

ACKNOWLEDGEMENT

Declared none.

REFERENCES

[1]   Weir HK, Thompson TD, Soman A, Møller B, Leadbetter S. The past, present, and future of cancer incidence in the United States: 1975 through 2020. Cancer 2015; 121(11): 1827-37.
[http://dx.doi.org/10.1002/cncr.29258] [PMID: 25649671]

[2]   Zhang C, Zhang C, Wang Q, Li Z, Lin J, Wang H. Differences in stage of cancer at diagnosis, treatment, and survival by race and ethnicity among leading cancer types. JAMA Netw Open 2020; 3(4): e202950.
[http://dx.doi.org/10.1001/jamanetworkopen.2020.2950] [PMID: 32267515]

[3]   Walsh S, *et al.* Decision support systems in oncology. JCO Clinical Cancer Informatics 2019; 3: 1-9.
[http://dx.doi.org/10.1200/CCI.18.00001]

[4]   Huang S, Yang J, Fong S, Zhao Q. Mining prognosis index of brain metastases using artificial intelligence. Cancers (Basel) 2019; 11(8): E1140.
[http://dx.doi.org/10.3390/cancers11081140] [PMID: 31395825]

[5]   Abrahamian FM, *et al.* List of contributors. In: Cohen J, Powderly WG, Opal SM, Eds. Infectious Diseases. 4th ed. Elsevier 2017; pp. xv-xxxvi.
[http://dx.doi.org/10.1016/B978-0-7020-6285-8.00234-3]

[6]   Matter F. Infectious Diseases. 4th ed. Elsevier 2017; pp. i-ii.

[7]   Cohen J, Powderly WG, Opal SM, Eds. Copyright. Infectious Diseases. 4th ed. Elsevier 2017; p. iv.
[http://dx.doi.org/10.1016/B978-0-7020-6285-8.00274-4]

[8]   Cohen J, Powderly WG, Opal SM, Eds. Dedication. Infectious Diseases. 4th ed. Elsevier 2017; p. xxxvii.
[http://dx.doi.org/10.1016/B978-0-7020-6285-8.00277-X]

[9]   Somashekhar SP, Sepúlveda MJ, Puglielli S, *et al.* Watson for Oncology and breast cancer treatment recommendations: agreement with an expert multidisciplinary tumor board. Ann Oncol 2018; 29(2): 418-23.
[http://dx.doi.org/10.1093/annonc/mdx781] [PMID: 29324970]

[10]   Gao HX, Huang SG, Du JF, *et al.* Comparison of prognostic indices in NSCLC patients with brain metastases after radiosurgery. Int J Biol Sci 2018; 14(14): 2065-72.
[http://dx.doi.org/10.7150/ijbs.28608] [PMID: 30585269]

[11]   Bera K, Schalper KA, Rimm DL, Velcheti V, Madabhushi A. Artificial intelligence in digital pathology - new tools for diagnosis and precision oncology. Nat Rev Clin Oncol 2019; 16(11): 703-15.
[http://dx.doi.org/10.1038/s41571-019-0252-y] [PMID: 31399699]

[12]   Shortliffe EH, *et al.* An expert system for oncology protocol management. In: Buchanan BG, Shortiffe EH, Eds. Rule-Based Expert Systems. 1984; pp. 653-65.

[13]   Dix A. Human-computer interaction. In: Liu L, ÖZsu MT, Eds. Encyclopedia of Database Systems. Boston, MA.: Springer US 2009; pp. 1327-31.

[14]   Carroll JM. HCI models, theories, and frameworks: Toward a multidisciplinary science. Elsevier 2003.

[15]   Wang F-H, Shen L, Li J, *et al.* The chinese society of clinical oncology (CSCO): clinical guidelines for the diagnosis and treatment of gastric cancer. Cancer Commun (Lond) 2019; 39(1): 10.
[http://dx.doi.org/10.1186/s40880-019-0349-9] [PMID: 30885279]

[16]   Preece J, Sharp H, Rogers Y. Interaction design: beyond human-computer interaction. John Wiley & Sons 2015.

[17]   Burris HA III, Rugo HS, Vukelja SJ, *et al.* Phase II study of the antibody drug conjugate trastuzumab-DM1 for the treatment of human epidermal growth factor receptor 2 (HER2)-positive breast cancer after prior HER2-directed therapy. J Clin Oncol 2011; 29(4): 398-405.
[http://dx.doi.org/10.1200/JCO.2010.29.5865] [PMID: 21172893]

[18]   Rieber A, Brambs HJ, Gabelmann A, Heilmann V, Kreienberg R, Kühn T. Breast MRI for monitoring response of primary breast cancer to neo-adjuvant chemotherapy. Eur Radiol 2002; 12(7): 1711-9.
[http://dx.doi.org/10.1007/s00330-001-1233-x] [PMID: 12111062]

[19]   Schagen SB, van Dam FS, Muller MJ, Boogerd W, Lindeboom J, Bruning PF. Cognitive deficits after postoperative adjuvant chemotherapy for breast carcinoma. Cancer 1999; 85(3): 640-50.
[http://dx.doi.org/10.1002/(SICI)1097-0142(19990201)85:3<640::AID-CNCR14>3.0.CO;2-G] [PMID: 10091737]

[20]   Evens AM, Antillón M, Aschebrook-Kilfoy B, Chiu BC. Racial disparities in Hodgkin's lymphoma: a comprehensive population-based analysis. Ann Oncol 2012; 23(8): 2128-37.
[http://dx.doi.org/10.1093/annonc/mdr578] [PMID: 22241896]

[21]   Xiang C, *et al.* Towards continuous access control validation and forensics. Proceedings of the 2019 ACM SIGSAC Conference on Computer and Communications Security. 2019.
[http://dx.doi.org/10.1145/3319535.3363191]

[22]   Adegboyega TO, Landercasper J, Linebarger JH, *et al.* Institutional review of compliance with NCCN guidelines for breast cancer: lessons learned from real-time multidimensional synoptic reporting. J Natl Compr Canc Netw 2015; 13(2): 177-83.
[http://dx.doi.org/10.6004/jnccn.2015.0026] [PMID: 25691610]

[23]   Charles C, Gafni A, Whelan T. Decision-making in the physician-patient encounter: revisiting the shared treatment decision-making model. Soc Sci Med 1999; 49(5): 651-61.
[http://dx.doi.org/10.1016/S0277-9536(99)00145-8] [PMID: 10452420]

[24]   Khan S, Yairi T. A review on the application of deep learning in system health management. Mech Syst Signal Process 2018; 107: 241-65.
[http://dx.doi.org/10.1016/j.ymssp.2017.11.024]

[25]   Emanuel EJ, Emanuel LL. Four models of the physician-patient relationship. JAMA 1992; 267(16): 2221-6.
[http://dx.doi.org/10.1001/jama.1992.03480160079038] [PMID: 1556799]

[26]   Preece A, *et al.* Better knowledge management through knowledge engineering. IEEE Intell Syst 2001; 16(1): 36-43.
[http://dx.doi.org/10.1109/5254.912383]

[27]   Hu Q, Yang J, Qin P, Fong S. Towards a Context-Free Machine Universal Grammar (CF-MUG) in Natural Language Processing. IEEE Access 2020; 8: 165111-29.
[http://dx.doi.org/10.1109/ACCESS.2020.3022674]

[28]   Yang J, Huang SG, Tang R. Broad Learning with Attribute Selection for Rheumatoid Arthritis, in IEEE International Conference on Systems, Man and Cybernetics (SMC), IEEE, Toronto, 2020.

[29]   Hu Q, Yang J, Qin P, Fong S, Guo J. Could or could not of Grid-Loc: grid BLE structure for indoor localisation system using machine learning. Serv Oriented Comput Appl 2020.
[http://dx.doi.org/10.1007/s11761-020-00292-z]

[30]   Yang J, Fong S, Li T. Attribute reduction based on multi-objective decomposition-ensemble optimizer with rough set and entropy. International Conference on Data Mining Workshops (ICDMW). IEEE 2019; pp. 673-80.

[31]   Huang S, Yang J, Fong S, Zhao Q. Artificial intelligence in cancer diagnosis and prognosis: Opportunities and challenges. Cancer Lett 2020; 471: 61-71.
[http://dx.doi.org/10.1016/j.canlet.2019.12.007] [PMID: 31830558]

CHAPTER 5

Current Medical Imaging and Artificial Intelligence and its Future

Shigao Huang[1], Jie Yang[2,3], Lijian Tan[3], Simon Fong[2,4] and Qi Zhao[1]

[1] *Institute of Translational Medicine, Faculty of Health Sciences, University of Macau 999078, Macau SAR, China*

[2] *Department of Computer and Information Science, University of Macau, Macau, China*

[3] *Chongqing Industry & Trade Polytechnic, Chongqing, China*

[4] *Zhuhai Institutes of Advanced Technology of the Chinese Academy of Sciences, China*

Abstract: "Artificial intelligence and medical image" is an auxiliary tool for the computer to complete image classification, target detection, image segmentation, and retrieval and assist doctors in diagnosing and treatment based on medical image through deep learning. This chapter includes the review of Artificial intelligence (AI) and its application in radiology, pathology, eye disease, deontology, dermatology, and ophthalmology, which we have benefited from the use of AI methods. Modern medicine is evidence-based medicine based on experiments. Doctors' diagnosis and treatment conclusions must be based on corresponding diagnostic data. Imaging is an important part of diagnosing, and 80% to 90% of data in the medical industry are derived from medical imaging. Therefore, clinicians have a strong demand for images, and they need to conduct a variety of quantitative analyses of medical images and comparison of historical images to complete a diagnosis. In contrast to this qualitative reasoning, AI is good at identifying complex patterns in the data and providing quantitative assessments in an automated manner. Integrating AI into clinical workflows as a tool to assist physicians allows for more accurate and repeatable radiological assessments.

Keywords: Artificial intelligence, Deontology, Eye disease, Medical imaging, Radiological assessments.

1. INTRODUCTION

Medical fields that rely on imaging data include radiology, pathology, dermatology, and ophthalmology [1], which have been benefited from the use of

* **Corresponding author Shigao Huang:** Institute of Translational Medicine, Faculty of Health Sciences, University of Macau 999078, Macau SAR, China; Tel: 853 88222953; Fax: 853 88222953; E-mail: huangshigao2010@aliyun.com

AI methods. In radiology, for example, experienced physicians evaluate medical images visually to detect, characterize, and monitor the disease [2]. This assessment is usually based on personal experience and is subjective. In contrast to this qualitative reasoning, AI is good at identifying complex patterns in the data and providing quantitative assessments in an automated manner [3]. Fig. (**1**) shows AI to screen the medical imaging quickly to find the lesions in the mammography radiation photograph, which is a combination of technology with AI and GSM. Integrating AI into clinical workflows as a tool to assist physicians allows for more accurate and repeatable radiological assessments.

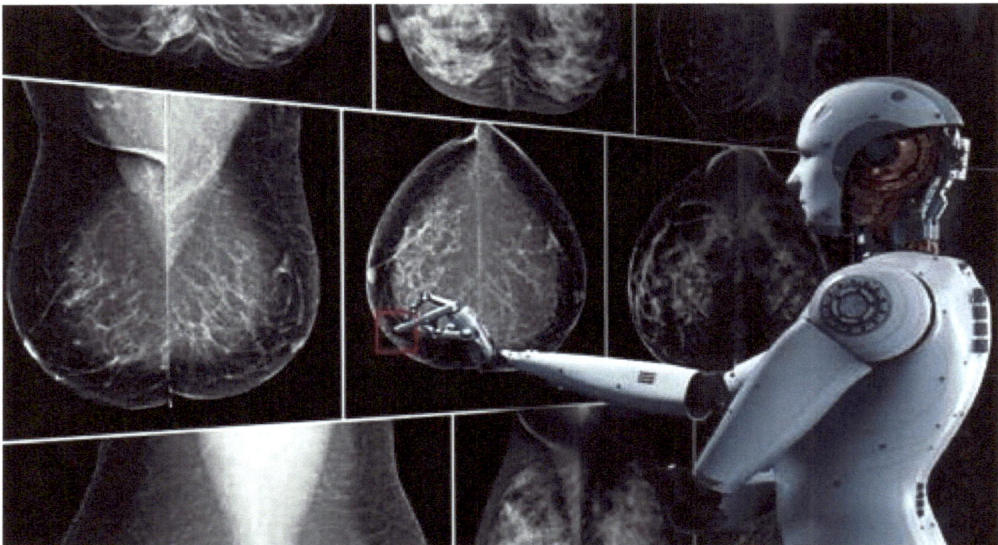

Fig. (1). National Cancer Institute sends AI to make smarter mammography. AI mammogram" is a combination of technology with AI and GSM. The purpose of the National Cancer Institute is to extend breast cancer prevention, help to speed up the service, reduce the workload of the staff, which can also help in reducing the costs and increasing the opportunities for Thais to access the service. (Source:https://newsbeezer.com/thailandeng/national-cancer-institute-sends-ai-t--make-smarter-mammography/).

At present, two kinds of AI methods are widely used in medical images. The first is artificial feature engineering, in which features are defined by mathematical equations, such as tumor textures, and can be quantified by a computer program. These artificial features serve as inputs to machine learning models trained to classify patients using clinical decision-making [4]. Although these characteristics are different, they rely on expert definitions and are therefore not necessarily the best quantification of the characteristics currently being used to identify tasks. Besides, predefined features are generally not applicable to imaging model changes, such as computed tomography (CT), positron emission tomography (PET) [5], and magnetic resonance imaging (MRI), and their associated signal-to-noise ratio characteristics. The second approach, a deep learning algorithm, automatically learns feature representations from the data without intervention by human experts. This data-driven approach allows for more abstract feature definitions, making them more informative and generalizable. Therefore, deep learning can automatically quantify the phenotypic characteristics of human tissues and can make substantial progress in diagnosis and clinical care [6].

Another benefit of deep learning is that it reduces the need for artificial preprocessing. Like a trained radiologist, deep learning can identify image parameters and weigh their importance against other factors to make clinical decisions [7].

2. PROCESS OF AI IN MEDICAL IMAGING

At present, more than 90% of medical data is obtained from medical imaging, and medical imaging data has become one of the essential "pieces of evidence" for doctors in diagnosis. AI can be used to help doctors make an accurate diagnosis. In that case, it is the current direction of efforts of many imaging AI explorers, which is of great help to widely improve the accuracy of disease diagnosis and treatment [8]. The following are four steps to achieve AI application in medical imaging.

2.1. Develop Standardized Use Cases

According to a study, the cases of AI used in medical imaging lack the standard inputs and outputs as compared to the algorithms already in use. As the algorithm may need to run on a local server or cloud service, a standard method needs to be developed to accept the input and output processed by the algorithm. Moreover, without the standardized inputs and outputs for AI cases, training and testing to develop standard data sets become more challenging, thus resulting in the output algorithm showing different results for the same case [9].

Ideally, AI cases need to be developed in the same format that can translate human narrative descriptions of what an algorithm should do into machine-readable languages, such as extensible Markup Language (extensible Markup Language) or JavaScript object representation using well-defined data elements. According to a study, structured used cases can help AI algorithms create validation standards before they are ready for clinical use, and applications in medical imaging can help achieve those standards. Medical professionals, academic institutions, and radiologists in medical imaging have a positive impact on AI development, and they all need to be involved in this structured development used cases to create common standards and structures and build specific AI used cases [10]. These cases can help AI algorithms establish the same definitions and develop practicable clinical approaches [8].

2.2. Establish a Data Sharing Method

To develop high-performance AI algorithms, models will need to learn from high-quality data sets that contain appropriate annotations or rich metadata. While there has been a lot of innovation around the topic, according to the study, it was mainly available in data-rich organizations only and these issues could limit the wide availability of information. Privacy concerns will limit the disclosure of patient data by such institutions, and these conditions will hinder the development of AI. Expediting the release of publicly available data sets and helping AI to be applied more quickly in clinical practice, and ensuring that patient data is used in a way that ensures its safety so that more diverse data are available, is critical.

2.3. Assess Clinical Practice and Infrastructure Needs

As per the report, the current lack of user interfaces in AI algorithms in clinical workflows limits the widespread use of AI models in clinical settings. IT developers need to create an efficient user interface and user experience design so that AI can be integrated with existing clinical workflow tools to accelerate the use of AI. Besides, developers need to establish vendor-neutral interoperability standards for communications between healthy IT systems. Understanding infrastructure needs, including qualitative and quantitative analysis of how AI will be deployed in clinical practice - whether local or cloud-based - will be key for the thousands of AI algorithms that can be used in real clinical practice. The medical imaging community must involve in assessing clinical practice and infrastructure needs and work with existing standards bodies, such as the National Science Foundation and the NIH Connected Health Initiative, to find solutions that can contribute to the adoption of AI in clinical practice.

2.4. Ensure Technical Safety and Accuracy

According to the study healthcare, stakeholders should work with IT developers, government agencies, and public organizations to ensure the accuracy of AI algorithms, reduce unconscious bias, and keep patients safe. To do this, stakeholders need to use data sets that contain demographic and technological diversity to validate AI algorithms. Federal agencies, such as the FDA need to play a key role in validating AI models to ensure patient safety. According to the report, FDA supervises a wide range of medical imaging devices, computer-aided diagnostic software, and other algorithms to support decision making for healthcare practitioners. The agency has long recognized the rapid growth of digitization across the health care sector, as well as the importance of regulating computer software that can detect and classify disease processes. Since 2012, It has been issuing regulatory guidance for software computer-aided testing and computer-aided diagnosis. Clinicians in the field of medical imaging will be the key to advancing cross-industry cooperation. Creating models for the validation and monitoring of AI algorithms and minimizing unconscious bias will require collaboration between researchers, industry developers, and government agencies. The medical imaging community should play a leading role in promoting these collaborations.

Although there are many obstacles to overcome, the application of AI in medical imaging is promising. In the future, industry stakeholders will need to work together to ensure that technology is safe, effective, and efficient. There are great prospects for AI applications in improving diagnosis and image-based diagnosis. The opportunities and challenges summarized here can serve as a roadmap for future development.

3. APPLICATION OF AI + MEDICAL IMAGING IN VARIOUS FIELDS

There are three main applications of AI in the field of medical imaging, namely disease screening, lesion delineation, and three-dimensional imaging of viscera.

We summarized the main coverage methods and types of medical images used by AI in medical imaging. Next, we will introduce the application of AI in lung screening, sugar mesh screening, lesion delineation, three-dimensional imaging of viscera, and pathological analysis, which are the most popular at present.

3.1. Lung Screening

The steps for AI to perform lung screening are as follows: image segmentation algorithm is used to process the lung scan sequence, generate the lung area map, and then generate the lung image based on the lung area map. The pulmonary region image generated by the pulmonary segmentation and the nodule labeling information was used to generate the nodule region image. The pulmonary nodule segmenting device based on the convolutional neural network was trained, and then the pulmonary nodules were segmented from the image to obtain the suspected pulmonary nodules. After the suspected pulmonary nodules are found, the 3D convolutional neural network is used to classify the pulmonary nodules, to obtain the location and confidence of the real pulmonary nodules.

3.2. Screening for Radiculopathy

Sugar mesh disease is the abbreviation of "diabetic retinopathy". It is a common retinal vascular disease and the main cause of blindness in diabetic patients. As sugar mesh disease does not have any clinical symptoms very often, but once symptoms start to appear, the disease becomes severe, and the best time for treatment is already missed. Therefore, the therapeutic effect of sugar mesh disease depends upon whether the treatment is timely or not. However, due to the shortage of ophthalmologists in China and the low attention of residents, the proportion of screening for sugar grid disease in China is less than 10% at present.

3.3. Target Outline

Target delineation and treatment plan design occupy a lot of time for oncologists. When patients are diagnosed with tumors, they tend to be panic and ask the doctor if there is any slightest movement in the body. However, the oncology department of the famous Grade three to Grae one hospitals is usually overcrowded. Besides visiting doctors, doctors are also involved in other tasks such as scientific research, *etc*. When they face endless questions from patients, they get irritated [11]. Oncologists in primary medical institutions are inexperienced, and in many cases, they are afraid to make treatment plans for patients, so they can only refer patients, which exacerbates the contradiction between doctors and patients in grade three hospitals. Therefore, it is of great concern for hospitals to use new technologies to improve the efficiency of doctors, improve the treatment level and confidence of primary doctors. In the process of tumor treatment, two tasks occupy a lot of doctors' time and energy. They are target area delineation and treatment plan design, respectively.

3.4. Three-dimensional Imaging of Viscera

Three-dimensional (3-D) imaging of Viscera is an AI-based data of medical images, such as MRI and CT, to locate and segment the target viscera and display the internal situation of the patient on the computer. The patient's MRI, CT, and other disease image data on the computer, display the patient's internal situation [12]. The probe in the doctor's hand points to the system updates and displays in real-time, allowing the doctor to have a clear understanding of the patient's anatomical location, making the surgical operation faster, more accurate, and safer.

3.5. Pathological Analysis

Even highly trained pathologists have different diagnoses for the same patient, and this difference is an important cause of misdiagnosis. For example, doctors' diagnoses of some forms of breast and prostate cancer were as low as 48 percent consistent. The lack of consistency shown by the doctors is not surprising. To make an accurate diagnosis, doctors must judge the amount of information available. Normally, the pathologist is responsible for reviewing all the biological tissue visible on the biopsy, but each patient has many biopsies, each of which has over 10 billion pixels (10+gigapixels) after 40 times magnification.

We reviewed the literature on the application of AI to the prognosis of various cancers in different research populations by scientists around the world (Table **1**). In the past decade, the number of such studies has increased rapidly in China, the United States, and Europe. Generally, medical statistics covers methods such as the area under the curve (AUC). Cancer prognosis involves the recurrence of the disease and the survival of the patient, and its purpose is to improve patient management. Bychkov *et al.* [41] trained a classifier based on deep learning to predict the five-year survival rate for specific diseases in a series of digitized tumor tissue samples stained for CRC, which require basic morphological staining, and the level of TMA points and the entire slide was performed by human experts. Compared with experienced human observers, b) Haenssle *et al.* [62] aims to promote the detection of melanoma. These levels are divided into the following categories: Level I only involves dermoscopy. Therefore, doctors with different levels of training and experience can benefit by using CNN's image classification capabilities.

Table 1. AI applied to various kinds of cancer prognosis by the global scientist in the different study population.

Type of Cancer	Authors	Year	Country/ Region	Number of Patients in Study	Study Population	Methods	Results
Breast Cancer	Sun *et al* [24]	2018	China	1980		Multimodal DNN	/
	Park *et al* [25]	2013	USA	162500	SEER	Semi-supervised Learning Model	/
	Delen *et al* [26]	2005	USA	433272	SEER	ANN and DT	Accuracy: DT (93.6%), ANN (91.2%)
	Lu *et al* [27]	2019	USA	82707	SEER	Dynamic Gradient Boosting Machine with GA	Accuracy Improved (28%)
	Samala *et al* [28]	2018	USA	2566	Both	DCNN	AUC(0.85±0.05)

(Table 1) cont.....

Type of Cancer	Authors	Year	Country/ Region	Number of Patients in Study	Study Population	Methods	Results
Gastric Cancer	Biglarian *et al* [29]	2011	Iran	436	Hospital	Cox Proportional Hazard, ANN	TP(83.1%),
	Zhu *et al* [30]	2013	China	289	Hospital	ANN	TP: ANN(85.3%)
	Zhu *et al* [31]	2019	China	203	Hospital	CNN	Sensitivity(76.47%), and Specificity(95.56%), Overall Accuracy(89.16%),CI(95%,90-97)
Glioblastoma	Vasudevan *et al* [32]	2018	India	215	TCGA	Neural Network	Accuracy: DT (89.2%)
Bladder Cancer	Tian *et al* [33]	2019	China	115	Hospital	Statistical Analysis	NEDD8: Poor Prognosis Found
	Hasnain *et al* [34]	2019	USA	3503	Hospital	KNN, RF, *etc*	Sensitivity& Specificity (>70%)
Nasopharyngeal Carcinoma	Zhang *et al* [35]	2019	China	3269	Hospital	Large Scale, Big Data Intelligence Platform	EBV DNA: a Robust Biomarker for NPC Prognosis
Prostate Cancer	Kuo *et al* [36]	2015	Taiwan	100	Hospital	Fuzzy Neural Network	/
	Zhang *et al* [37]	2017	USA	/	TCGA	SVM model	Average Accuracy (66%)
	Stephan *et al* [38]	2002	Germany	928	Hospital	ANN	Specificity Level(90%)
Colorectal Cancer	Bottaci *et al* [39]	1997	UK	334	Hospital	Six Neural Networks	Accuracy(>80%), mean Sensitivity(60%), mean Specificity(88%)
	Wang *et al* [40]	2019	China	1568	SEER	Semi-random Regression Tree	/
	Bychkov *et al* [41]	2018	Finland	641	Hospital	LSTM, Naïve Bayes, SVM	Hazard Ratio(2.3); CI(95%,1.79–3.03), AUC(0.69)
Oral Cancer	Chang *et al* [42]	2013	Malaysia	156	MOCDTBS	Hybrid model of ReliefF-GA-ANFIS	Accuracy (93.81%), AUC (0.9)
Lung Cancer	Lynch *et al* [43]	2017	USA	10442	SEER	GBM, SVM	RMSE(32,15.05) for GBM, SVM
	Sepehri *et al* [44]	2018	France	101	Hospital	SVM with RFE and RF	Accuracy(71%, 59%)
	Yu *et al* [45]	2016	Italy	168	Hospital	Naive Bayes, SVM with Gaussian, *etc*	/
Ovarian Cancer	Lu *et al* [46]	2019	Taiwan	84	Both	SVM	HR(0.644), CI(95%,0.436-0.952)
	Lu *et al* [47]	2019	UK	364	Both	Unsupervised Hierarchical Clustering	RPV: A Novel Prognostic Signature Discovered
	Acharya *et al* [48]	2018	Singapore& Malaysia	469	Hospital	Fuzzy Forest	Accuracy(80.60 ± 0.5%), Sensitivity(81.40%), Specificity (76.30%)

(Table 1) cont.....

Type of Cancer	Authors	Year	Country/ Region	Number of Patients in Study	Study Population	Methods	Results
Glioma	Lu *et al* [49]	2018	Taiwan	456	TCGA	Improved SVM	Accuracy(81.8%), ROC(0.922)
	Papp *et al* [50]	2018	Austria	70	Hospital	GA and Nelder–Mead ML methods	Sensitivity (86%-98%), Specificity (92%-95%)
Spinal Chordoma	Karhade *et al* [51]	2018	USA	265	SEER	Boosted DT, SVM, ANN	5-year Survival (67.5%)
Long Bone Metastases	Stein *et al* [52]	2015	USA	927	Hospital	Multiple Additive Regression Trees	/
Oral Cavity Squamous Cell	Lu *et al* [53]	2017	USA	115	Hospital	RF, SVM	AUC(0.72), Accuracy(70.77), Specificity(73.08), Sensitivity(61.54)
Pancreatic Neuroendocrine	Song *et al* [54]	2018	China	8422	SEER	SVM, RF, DL	Accuracy(81.6%±1.9%),curve(0.87)
Thyroid cancer	Li *et al* [55]	2019	China	17627	Both	DCNN	Sensitivity (93.4%), CI (95%,89.6-96.1) Specificity (86.1%,p<0.0001)
Skin cancer	Esteva *et al* [56]	2017	USA	2032	Both	Inception v3 CNN	AUC(over 91%)
Non-small cell lung cancer	Coudray *et al* [57]	2018	USA	137	TCGA, NCI Genomic Data Commons	DCNN(inception v3)	AUC(0.733-0.856)
Non-small cell lung cancer	Wu *et al* [58]	2018	Italy	1034	Hospital	Bayesian network	/
Non-Hodgkin's lymphomas	Lorenzo *et al* [59]	1999	Italy	98	Hospital	Multivariate Cluster Analysis	/
Breast Invasive Ductal Carcinoma	Nadia *et al* [60]	2019	Italy	374	Lymphoma and IDC Datasets	Convolutional Autoencoder, Supervised Encoder FusionNet	F-measure Score Improved(5.06%), Accuracy Improved(5.06%)
Pan-Renal Cell Carcinoma	Tabibu *et al* [61]	2019	India	Ensemble	TCGA	CNN	Accuracy(92.61%)
Dermoscopic melanoma	Haenssle *et al* [62]	2018	International Skin Imaging Collaboration (ISIC)	100	International Skin Imaging Collaboration (ISIC)	Google's Inception v4 CNN architecture	Sensitivities(86.6%-88.9%, ROC AUC(>0.86,P < 0.01)

*SVM: Support Vector Machine, DNN: Deep Neural Network, ANN: Artificial Neural Network, DT: Decision Tree, GA: Genetic Algorithm Optimizer, KNN: K-Nearest Neighbor, RF: Random Forest, LSTM: Long Short-Term Memory Network, GBM: Gradient Boosting Machines, RFE: Recursive Feature Elimination, TP: True Prediction; AUC: Area Under the Curve, Ensemble:1027 (KIRC), 303 (KIRP), and 254 (KICH) tumor slide image. (Table **1** was cited and merged from my previous study and obtained approval. Huang *et al*. 2019).

4. AI AND ITS APPLICATIONS IN EYE DISEASE

Blood vessel segmentation techniques in fundus image analysis and computer-aided diagnosis in various eye diseases play an important role in the current medical practice. It is the foundation of medical diagnosis, surgery-aided design, and for early detection and treatment of various cardiovascular diseases and eye diseases [13] which include stroke, venous congestion, diabetes retinopathy, and hardening of the arteries.

In recent years, vascular segmentation has become one of the hot issues in the field of medical imaging. Many automatic segmentation techniques have been proposed and these have achieved good results (Fig. **2**). AI diagnosis system for eye diseases has been established *via* Ultra-wide-angle. However, as an auxiliary technology, the image matting model is rarely applied in vascular segmentation. So far, we have only found one patent, which performs vascular segmentation by invariant moment feature and KNN matting technology. However, since generating Trimap is a tedious and time-consuming task in the process of vascular segmentation, it is necessary to design an appropriate image matting algorithm to segment vessels as efficiently as possible.

The process of vascular segmentation algorithm based on the hierarchical Matting model consists of Trimap Generation and Matting. In the generation of trisomy, to improve the contrast of blood vessels, we use wavelet transform and morphological processing to enhance the overall features of blood vessels, and then combine threshold processing and shape features of blood vessels to realize image segmentation and arterial trunk extraction, to obtain trisomy of fundus images.

5. AI IN DENTISTRY

5.1. The Rise of Machine Learning

Big data sets are needed to train smart systems [14]. The project uses deep learning to extract meaning from 10m YouTube video images. Amazingly, Machine learning is the most advanced technology in the field of AI. Dentists now have an in-depth learning AI platform to detect cavities. AI, in the later stages of clinical evaluation, allows any licensed dentist to register as an investigator and use the system.

5.2. The Future of AI in Dentistry

When you hear about AI, you might think of science fiction and imagination, but the future of AI in dentistry is bright [15]. Some of us remember Will Robinson's loyal robot friend from the Lost In Space series of the 1960s. Others will trace the sci-fi vision of intelligent autonomous robots back to the day in the Terminator films when Skynet's sense of self and humanity began. The term AI and the scientific community's official pursuit of intelligent machines dates back to the Dartmouth and IBM conference of researchers in 1956. The use of AI in the dental field has emerged! It was easy for the dentist to check for cavities with an X-ray. We have read radiology in practice for thousands of years. Even so, it is estimated that x-rays may misdiagnose cavities. Radiologists must be "trained" to recognize meaningful patterns. They must be able to understand new information in the form of spoken, written text, or images, with appropriate context and nuance.

Finally, they must be able to make decisions based on new information and then learn from their mistakes to improve their decision-making process. For AI systems to have any real benefit in the real world, all of this must happen at the same time that humans perform the same tasks. Until recently, large-scale adoption of AI was not technically feasible or cost-effective, so the reality of AI has not matched the possibilities. Whatever the technical challenges may be, machines do offer some clear advantages. Computers are not biased. As human beings, we are naturally biased and we may make judgments too early. The computer considers only the data provided. Machines don't get tired. We can work for four or five hours without getting tired; the machine works 24 hours a day with no breaks. Another advantage is that machines don't get bored. The tasks we are happy to unload are monotonous and repetitive. Finally, the machine is fast. While current AI systems are primarily based on training and programming for specific tasks (for example, reading radiological images and predicting the location of cavities), they are generally much faster than humans.

Overall, the US Food and Drug Administration started making developments began two years ago. However, significant progress has been made in providing predictive assistants [16]. AI evaluated systems outperform dentists in "sensitivity" by accurately predicting the proportion of cavities that, in reality, the total number of caries is real. Although the machine matched the accuracy of one of the three dentists, the dentist won the title for "accuracy" -In the next 12 to 24 months, AI may emerge, as an application to detect periodontal disease and bone loss associated with periodontal disease [17].

The use of AI in dentistry will spread rapidly in the next years to come. In the next 10 to 15 years, the use of AI-based technologies in practice will be as common and pervasive as practice management and imaging systems are today.

6. EFFECTS OF AI ON TUMOR IMAGE WORKFLOW

There are three main clinical, radiographic tasks in oncology: anomaly detection, characterization, and change monitoring. In the workflow of manual anomaly detection, radiologists can identify possible anomalies based on personal experience. Dependence on computers or computer-aided detection (CAD) can misguide physicians to make abnormal detection (Fig. **2**) [18 - 19]; For example, the traditional image of PET-CT and AI platform to diagnose disease is shown in Fig. (**3**). Recent studies have shown that CAD based on deep learning is superior to CAD systems with traditional artificial features and that human performance is similar [10]. Characterization is a general term covering disease segmentation, diagnosis, and staging. The most recent deep learning architecture used for segmentation includes the fully convolutional network, which only includes the convolutional layer and the output in the segmentation probability graph of the whole image. Other architectures, such as U-NET, are specifically designed for medical imaging.

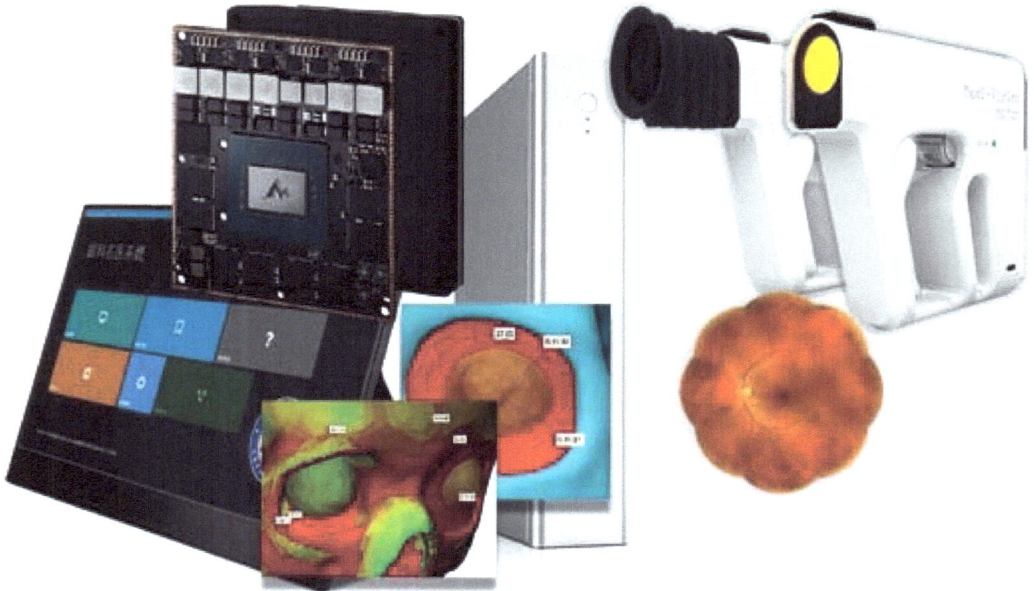

Fig. (2). Ultra-wide-angle AI diagnosis system for eye diseases.

Tumor radiation image feature including size, maximum diameter, the spherical degree, internal texture and edge definition of information, *etc.*, are the characteristics to determine the diagnosis of a benign and malignant tumor, which is often subjective, but architecture like CNN, due to the automatic feature extraction, is very suitable for supervision and diagnosis. The staging system divides patients into predefined categories by segmenting and diagnosing before information gathering. Disease surveillance is essential for diagnosis and evaluation of treatment response. The workflow involves image registration processing, first aligning images from multiple scans of diseased tissue and then evaluating them using predefined metrics.

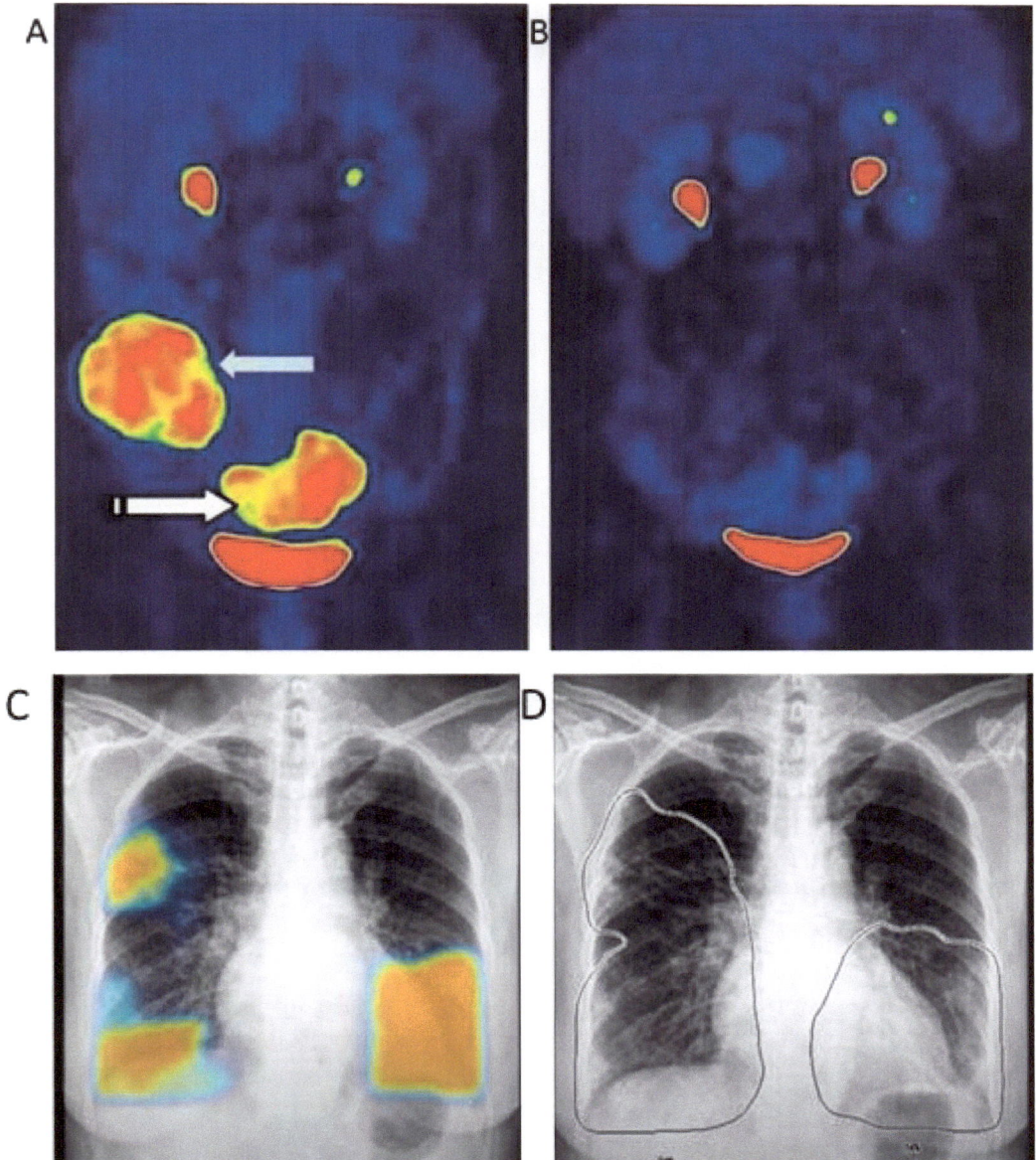

Fig. (3). Traditional image of PET-CT and AI platform to diagnose disease (A and B were cited from my previous study. Dang *et al*. 2018).

7. THE EXPLORATION AND DEVELOPMENT OF AI IMAGE

The following are summarized fourteen kinds of AI platform applications in medical imaging.

7.1. Philips

Intelligent tumor interventional treatment applied Onco Suite is the industry's first tumor comprehensive plan, tumor embolism, and percutaneous ablation to provide a one-stop solution. It can optimize the tumor lesion, guide catheter in place, curative effect evaluation, and so on, making the treatment of big tumor treatment more thorough. At the same time, it helps in avoiding similar healthy tissue damage.

7.2. Ali Health

The "Doctor You" AI system of intelligent image diagnosis jointly developed by Ali Health and Wanliyun includes a scientific research diagnosis platform, medically assisted detection engine, physician ability training system, *etc.* Doctor, You's CT lung nodule intelligent detection engine is jointly built by Ali Health's algorithm engine team and Alibaba iDST's vision computing team. It combines medical knowledge and AI technology to automatically identify and mark suspicious nodules, improve doctors' efficiency, and reduce the rate of misdiagnosis.

7.3. Tencent Miying

Tencent Miying AI medical imaging connects medical experts, AI, and product support teams. It also integrates leading technologies in image recognition and deep learning with medicine to assist doctors in early cancer screening.

At present, Tencent Miying's AI auxiliary diagnostic ability mainly includes diagnosis, treatment risk monitoring system, and intelligent medical record management system: diagnosis and treatment risk monitoring system is designed to help reduce doctors' diagnosis and treatment risk.

The structural output of medical records can free doctors from the tedious superficial work of medical records and effectively improve the efficiency of diagnosis, treatment, and scientific research.

7.4. Hainer Medical Trust

Susquehanna medical aortic dissection and complete quantitative analysis system, for the blood vessels image segmentation algorithm, were based on AI and the automation of quantitative modeling algorithm. By employing this, in 5 minutes, the clinicians can establish the precise aortic vascular quantitative model for critical patients with aortic dissection. Thus it greatly improves the efficiency of disease diagnosis and interventional treatment of aortic dissection.

7.5. Deduce Technology

It is assumed that technological intelligent CT-assisted screening products not only improve the efficiency of lung cancer screening but also show superior sensitivity to semi-solid and ground glass nodules and other signs of early lung cancer, which can help radiologists to improve the accuracy of diagnosis and achieve technical breakthroughs in early diagnosis and treatment of lung cancer.

Its intelligent X-ray-assisted screening product can judge more than 20 different lesions in the thoracic region, which can not only help the doctor to quickly screen out the image of existing lesions but also can quickly identify the location of lesions in the diagnosis process of outpatient and inpatient cases.

7.6. Yassen Technologies

Using the original patent mathematical model, Yassen has carried out scientific research cooperation projects of quantitative analysis of brain, heart, lung, thyroid, and other organs with several key hospitals in China developed and verified the biological and mathematical analysis of specific diseases, and continuously established the database of normal people of China. Yassen's product is developed based on the SPM Statistical Parametric Mapping theory. SPM theory is mainly applied to the quantitative analysis of brain images, and the application of this theory is extended to the lungs, thyroid, and so on by Jason technology.

7.7. Hui-Yi Hui Ying

Hui-Yi huiying used AI to build a smart image cloud platform, aiming to improve the efficiency and accuracy of doctors' diagnosis and treatment and solve the problem of mismatch of doctor-patient resources in some regions. The accuracy of the automatic diagnosis of pneumothorax, tuberculosis, and mass on a chest X-ray has reached 95%. The automatic recognition rate of the tumor was over 85%. The recognition rate of pulmonary nodules in chest CT is over 85%.

7.8. Tuma Depth

Based on the deep learning technology, Tuma Depth's "Lung nodules Detection and Analysis System" can analyze chest CT thin-layer scan images, to help doctors examine and mark patients' lung nodules. Besides, it can also make benign and malignant judgments and automatically generate structured reports.

Compared with traditional artificial screening, this analysis system has great advantages in intelligence and efficiency. With the deep learning analysis system, the machine can automatically detect nodules, calculate various relevant parameters, automatically generate monitoring reports, and provide a reference for doctors.

7.9. Diyinjia

Inga team specializes in providing AI-based medical image big data analysis solutions for precision medicine, such as cancer diagnosis and classification based on pathological image analysis. Its main products include AI-assisted diagnosis systems and digital pathological remote consultation systems, *etc.*, which can process and analyze full-field scanning digital pathological images with data size over 1G in 5-10 seconds on ordinary computers. Meanwhile, the accuracy rate of benign and malignant discrimination of several kinds of cancers is up to over 98%. The model and algorithm developed by the Yinga team can accurately, quickly, and intelligently analyze the various medical images, calculate key index parameters, generate automatic data analysis and reports, and provide pathologists with intelligent diagnostic systems for 7 types of cancer, such as breast cancer, gastric cancer, and prostate cancer.

7.10. Heart Link Medical

Defiled the remote medical care, tumor treatment platform can be seamlessly connected to the existing commercial linear accelerators, for cancer patients to provide more accurate, more automatic, more rapid personalized clinical radiotherapy plan, to improve the cure rate of radiotherapy for cancer, reduce the radiation injury of normal tissue, ultimately prolong the life of cancer patients, and improve the quality of life of cancer patients. The system provides functions including target area delineation, data storage, and backup, cloud computing and sharing, image deformation registration, workflow management, and remote consultation.

7.11. DeepCare

Taking a page out of the SaaS playbook, DeepCare puts the developed smart modules for different diseases on the cloud platform, allowing device manufacturers and telemedicine providers to choose and pay for them according to their needs.

As it is in the early stages of data accumulation, DeepCare is willing to pay for the service by providing images.

7.12. Peptide Building Blocks

Starting from medical image-assisted reading, the research field of fundus lesions was first selected to carry out the screening and diagnosis of sugar mesh disease by analyzing fundus color photos.

The assistant diagnosis of glaucoma and other eye diseases is also continuously advancing. Peptide Blocks is cooperating with Zhong Shan Ophthalmology Department in Guangzhou to carry out research and development.

This AI application can mark the focus, auxiliary diagnosis, and generate medical records. It will mark the focus point, inform the doctor what the probability of a certain disease is, and provide treatment strategies, disease development prediction, *etc*. Treatment strategies may be either further review or direct intervention, such as drug therapy.

7.13. Smart Shadow Medical

The first phase of Smart medical products, based on radiological imaging and pathological imaging, provides two auxiliary diagnostic solutions, including the intelligent diagnostic system for early lung cancer, tuberculosis, and silicosis, and the cardiopulmonary health index analysis and management system for the general examination.

Based on intelligent diagnostic pathology image solutions, it has now launched automatically based on sputum microscopy imaging of pulmonary tuberculosis disease diagnosis system; it is using dyeing pathological picture image, combined with the depth study of the artificial neural network, cluster analysis, multi-resolution, boundary identification and fuzzy logic algorithm for cell pathological condition of regional image segmentation, image feature extraction and use of multi-stage classification treatment to accurately identify the pathological cells number and level.

7.14. Imagemesh Laboratory

Through computer vision technology and deep learning algorithms, the ImageBiopsy will help doctors to make accurate diagnoses based on the radiographs. Based on the NVIDIA GPU, the company trains its algorithm with more than 150,000 radiological images so that doctors can get accurate measurements of the knee circumference. Doctors can determine the severity of osteoarthritis based on the measurements without further diagnosis.

8. THE NEXT FRONTIER

As technological barriers fall and research shifts, we are certainly close to the threshold of providing a range of AI tools to dentistry. We have seen recent product introductions incorporating elements of AI and machine learning (AI/ML). A device, launched at the Midwinter Conference in Chicago, is an amazing technology supported by Natural Language Processing (NLP) [20]. Simplifier's digital assistant, developed with Simplifier, replaces the traditional point-to-point interface with simple, fast voice commands, scheduling optimization project called MMG Chair Fill [21] was also recently announced. The project treatments initiate new profit-maximizing algorithm-based patient marketing campaigns.

We will continue to see the rapid adoption of AI in areas of practice management and growth. With the latest capabilities of deep learning technology, AI will begin to affect dentistry on a clinical level. The first-hand experience of the technology at the development stage, for example, has demonstrated the potential value of AI [22].

We can foresee images from deep learning analysis tools to assist in the diagnosis. The detection and early intervention of implant periodontitis is a possible benefit of implant dentistry [22, 23]. It certainly will, in the future, provide more clinical decisions, making a better dentist. Here there is a long way to go to popularise this technology.

CONSENT FOR PUBLICATION

Not Applicable.

CONFLICT OF INTEREST

The author confirms that this chapter contents have no conflict of interest.

ACKNOWLEDGEMENT

Declared none.

REFERENCES

[1]   Hosny A, Parmar C, Quackenbush J, Schwartz LH, Aerts HJWL. Artificial intelligence in radiology. Nat Rev Cancer 2018; 18(8): 500-10.
[http://dx.doi.org/10.1038/s41568-018-0016-5] [PMID: 29777175]

[2]   Zhou LQ, Wang JY, Yu SY, *et al.* Artificial intelligence in medical imaging of the liver. World J Gastroenterol 2019; 25(6): 672-82.
[http://dx.doi.org/10.3748/wjg.v25.i6.672] [PMID: 30783371]

[3]   Bini SA. Artificial intelligence, machine learning, deep learning, and cognitive computing: what do these terms mean and how will they impact health care? J Arthroplasty 2018; 33(8): 2358-61.
[http://dx.doi.org/10.1016/j.arth.2018.02.067] [PMID: 29656964]

[4]   Kapoor R, Walters SP, Al-Aswad LA. The current state of artificial intelligence in ophthalmology. Surv Ophthalmol 2019; 64(2): 233-40.
[http://dx.doi.org/10.1016/j.survophthal.2018.09.002] [PMID: 30248307]

[5]   Vaquero JJ, Kinahan P. Positron emission tomography: current challenges and opportunities for technological advances in clinical and preclinical imaging systems. Annu Rev Biomed Eng 2015; 17: 385-414.
[http://dx.doi.org/10.1146/annurev-bioeng-071114-040723] [PMID: 26643024]

[6]   Uddin M, Wang Y, Woodbury-Smith M. Artificial intelligence for precision medicine in neurodevelopmental disorders. npj Digital Medicine 2019; 2(1): 112.

[7]   Liu K-L, Wu T, Chen PT, *et al.* Deep learning to distinguish pancreatic cancer tissue from non-cancerous pancreatic tissue: a retrospective study with cross-racial external validation. Lancet Digit Health 2020; 2(6): e303-13.
[http://dx.doi.org/10.1016/S2589-7500(20)30078-9] [PMID: 33328124]

[8]   Thrall JH, Li X, Li Q, *et al.* Artificial intelligence and machine learning in radiology: opportunities, challenges, pitfalls, and criteria for success. J Am Coll Radiol 2018; 15 (3 Pt B): 504-8.
[http://dx.doi.org/10.1016/j.jacr.2017.12.026] [PMID: 29402533]

[9]   Suzuki K. Overview of deep learning in medical imaging. Radiological Phys Technol 2017; 10(3): 257-73.
[http://dx.doi.org/10.1007/s12194-017-0406-5] [PMID: 28689314]

[10]   Allen B, Seltzer SE, Langlotz CP, *et al.* A Road map for translational research on artificial intelligence in medical imaging: From the 2018 national institutes of health/rsna/acr/the academy workshop. J Am Coll Radiol 2019; 16 (9 Pt A): 1179-89.
[http://dx.doi.org/10.1016/j.jacr.2019.04.014] [PMID: 31151893]

[11]   Reisdorf S. Artificial intelligence for the development of screening parameters in the field of corneal biomechanics. Klin Monatsbl Augenheilkd 2019; 236(12): 1423-7.
[PMID: 31805593]

[12]   Pesapane F, Codari M, Sardanelli F. Artificial intelligence in medical imaging: threat or opportunity? Radiologists again at the forefront of innovation in medicine. European Radiology Experimental 2018; 2(1): 35.
[http://dx.doi.org/10.1186/s41747-018-0061-6]

[13]   Whiting P, Rutjes AW, Reitsma JB, Glas AS, Bossuyt PM, Kleijnen J. Sources of variation and bias in studies of diagnostic accuracy: a systematic review. Ann Intern Med 2004; 140(3): 189-202.
[http://dx.doi.org/10.7326/0003-4819-140-3-200402030-00010] [PMID: 14757617]

[14]   Oussous A, *et al.* Big data technologies: A survey. J King Saud University - Computer and Information Sciences 2018; 30(4): 431-48.
[http://dx.doi.org/10.1016/j.jksuci.2017.06.001]

[15]   Hung K, Montalvao C, Tanaka R, Kawai T, Bornstein MM. The use and performance of artificial intelligence applications in dental and maxillofacial radiology: A systematic review. Dentomaxillofac Radiol 2020; 49(1): 20190107.
[http://dx.doi.org/10.1259/dmfr.20190107] [PMID: 31386555]

[16]   Fazal MI, Patel ME, Tye J, Gupta Y. The past, present and future role of artificial intelligence in imaging. Eur J Radiol 2018; 105: 246-50.
[http://dx.doi.org/10.1016/j.ejrad.2018.06.020] [PMID: 30017288]

[17]   Siegel E. Artificial intelligence and diagnostic radiology: Not quite ready to welcome our computer overlords. Appl Radiol 2012; 41(4): 8.

[18]   Dang YZ, Li X, Ma YX, *et al.* ^{18}F-FDG-PET/CT-guided intensity-modulated radiotherapy for 42 FIGO III/IV ovarian cancer: A retrospective study. Oncol Lett 2019; 17(1): 149-58.
[PMID: 30655750]

[19]   Chan HP, Hadjiiski LM, Samala RK. Computer-aided diagnosis in the era of deep learning. Med Phys 2020; 47(5): e218-27.
[http://dx.doi.org/10.1002/mp.13764] [PMID: 32418340]

[20]   Yin W, *et al.* Comparative study of cnn and rnn for natural language processing. ArXiv preprint arXiv:170201923 2017.

[21]   Masoleh BR. Utilizing Machine Learning and Virtual Reality to Facilitate Brain-Computer Interface Control. Canada: University of Toronto 2019.

[22]   Krupinski EA. The future of image perception in radiology: synergy between humans and computers. Acad Radiol 2003; 10(1): 1-3.
[http://dx.doi.org/10.1016/S1076-6332(03)80781-X] [PMID: 12529022]

[23]   Doi K. Computer-aided diagnosis in medical imaging: historical review, current status and future potential. Comput Med Imaging Graph 2007; 31(4-5): 198-211.
[http://dx.doi.org/10.1016/j.compmedimag.2007.02.002] [PMID: 17349778]

[24]   Sun D, Wang M, Li A. A multimodal deep neural network for human breast cancer prognosis prediction by integrating multi-dimensional data, IEEE/ACM Trans Comput Biol Bioinform, 2018.

[25]   Park K, Ali A, Kim D, An Y, Kim M, Shin H. Robust predictive model for evaluating breast cancer survivability. Eng Appl Artif Intell 2013; 26: 2194-205.
[http://dx.doi.org/10.1016/j.engappai.2013.06.013]

[26]   Delen D, Walker G, Kadam A. Predicting breast cancer survivability: a comparison of three data mining methods. Artif Intell Med 2005; 34(2): 113-27.
[http://dx.doi.org/10.1016/j.artmed.2004.07.002] [PMID: 15894176]

[27]   Lu H, Wang H, Yoon SW. A dynamic gradient boosting machine using genetic optimizer for practical breast cancer prognosis. Expert Syst Appl 2019; 116: 340-50.
[http://dx.doi.org/10.1016/j.eswa.2018.08.040]

[28]   Samala RK, Heang-Ping Chan , Hadjiiski L, Helvie MA, Richter CD, Cha KH. Breast cancer diagnosis in digital breast tomosynthesis: effects of training sample size on multi-stage transfer learning using deep neural nets. IEEE Trans Med Imaging 2019; 38(3): 686-96.
[http://dx.doi.org/10.1109/TMI.2018.2870343] [PMID: 31622238]

[29]   Biglarian A, Hajizadeh E, Kazemnejad A, Zali M. Application of artificial neural network in predicting the survival rate of gastric cancer patients. Iran J Public Health 2011; 40(2): 80-6.
[PMID: 23113076]

[30]   Zhu L, Luo W, Su M, *et al.* Comparison between artificial neural network and Cox regression model

in predicting the survival rate of gastric cancer patients. Biomed Rep 2013; 1(5): 757-60.
[http://dx.doi.org/10.3892/br.2013.140] [PMID: 24649024]

[31]   Zhu Y, Wang QC, Xu MD, *et al.* Application of convolutional neural network in the diagnosis of the invasion depth of gastric cancer based on conventional endoscopy Gastrointest Endosc ; 89(2019): 806-15. e801

[32]   Vasudevan P, Murugesan T. Cancer subtype discovery using prognosis-enhanced neural network classifier in multigenomic data. Technol Cancer Res Treat, 17 2018.

[33]   Tian DW, Wu ZL, Jiang LM, Gao J, Wu CL, Hu HL. Neural precursor cell expressed, developmentally downregulated 8 promotes tumor progression and predicts poor prognosis of patients with bladder cancer. Cancer Sci 2019; 110(1): 458-67.
[http://dx.doi.org/10.1111/cas.13865] [PMID: 30407690]

[34]   Hasnain Z, Mason J, Gill K, *et al.* Machine learning models for predicting post-cystectomy recurrence and survival in bladder cancer patients. PLoS One 2019; 14(2): e0210976.
[http://dx.doi.org/10.1371/journal.pone.0210976] [PMID: 30785915]

[35]   Zhang Y, Tang LL, Li YQ, Liu X, Liu Q, Ma J. Spontaneous remission of residual post-therapy plasma Epstein-Barr virus DNA and its prognostic implication in nasopharyngeal carcinoma: A large-scale, big-data intelligence platform-based analysis. Int J Cancer 2019; 144(9): 2313-9.
[http://dx.doi.org/10.1002/ijc.32021] [PMID: 30485420]

[36]   Kuo RJ, Huang MH, Cheng WC, Lin CC, Wu YH. Application of a two-stage fuzzy neural network to a prostate cancer prognosis system. Artif Intell Med 2015; 63(2): 119-33.
[http://dx.doi.org/10.1016/j.artmed.2014.12.008] [PMID: 25576196]

[37]   Zhang S, Xu Y, Hui X, *et al.* Improvement in prediction of prostate cancer prognosis with somatic mutational signatures. J Cancer 2017; 8(16): 3261-7.
[http://dx.doi.org/10.7150/jca.21261] [PMID: 29158798]

[38]   Stephan C, Jung K, Cammann H, *et al.* An artificial neural network considerably improves the diagnostic power of percent free prostate-specific antigen in prostate cancer diagnosis: results of a 5-year investigation. Int J Cancer 2002; 99(3): 466-73.
[http://dx.doi.org/10.1002/ijc.10370] [PMID: 11992419]

[39]   Bottaci L, Drew PJ, Hartley JE, *et al.* Artificial neural networks applied to outcome prediction for colorectal cancer patients in separate institutions. Lancet 1997; 350(9076): 469-72.
[http://dx.doi.org/10.1016/S0140-6736(96)11196-X] [PMID: 9274582]

[40]   Wang Y, Wang D, Ye X, Wang Y, Yin Y, Jin Y. A tree ensemble-based two-stage model for advanced-stage colorectal cancer survival prediction. Inf Sci 2019; 474: 106-24.
[http://dx.doi.org/10.1016/j.ins.2018.09.046]

[41]   Bychkov D, Linder N, Turkki R, *et al.* Deep learning based tissue analysis predicts outcome in colorectal cancer. Sci Rep 2018; 8(1): 3395.
[http://dx.doi.org/10.1038/s41598-018-21758-3] [PMID: 29467373]

[42]   Yang J, Huang SG, Tang R. Broad Learning with Attribute Selection for Rheumatoid Arthritis, in: IEEE International Conference on Systems, Man and Cybernetics (SMC), IEEE, Toronto, 2020.

[43]   Lynch CM, Abdollahi B, Fuqua JD, *et al.* Prediction of lung cancer patient survival *via* supervised machine learning classification techniques. Int J Med Inform 2017; 108: 1-8.
[http://dx.doi.org/10.1016/j.ijmedinf.2017.09.013] [PMID: 29132615]

[44]   Sepehri S, Upadhaya T, Desseroit M-C, Visvikis D, Le Rest CC, Hatt MJJNM. Comparison of machine learning algorithms for building prognostic models in non-small cell lung cancer using clinical and radiomics features from 18F-FDG PET/CT images. J Nucl Med 2018; 59: 328-8.

[45]   Yu KH, Zhang C, Berry GJ, *et al.* Predicting non-small cell lung cancer prognosis by fully automated microscopic pathology image features. Nat Commun 2016; 7: 12474.
[http://dx.doi.org/10.1038/ncomms12474] [PMID: 27527408]

[46] TP Lu, KT Kuo, CH Chen, MC Chang, HP Lin, YH Hu, YC Chiang, WF Cheng, CA Chen, Developing a Prognostic Gene Panel of Epithelial Ovarian Cancer Patients by a Machine Learning Model. Basel: Cancers 2019; p. 11.

[47] Lu H, Arshad M, Thornton A, *et al.* A mathematical-descriptor of tumor-mesoscopic-structure from computed-tomography images annotates prognostic- and molecular-phenotypes of epithelial ovarian cancer. Nat Commun 2019; 10(1): 764.
[http://dx.doi.org/10.1038/s41467-019-08718-9] [PMID: 30770825]

[48] Acharya UR, Akter A, Chowriappa P, *et al.* Use of nonlinear features for automated characterization of suspicious ovarian tumors using ultrasound images in fuzzy forest framework. Int J Fuzzy Systems 2018; 20: 1385-402.

[49] Lu CF, Hsu FT, Hsieh KL, *et al.* Machine learning-based radiomics for molecular subtyping of gliomas. Clin Cancer Res 2018; 24(18): 4429-36.
[http://dx.doi.org/10.1158/1078-0432.CCR-17-3445] [PMID: 29789422]

[50] Papp L, Pötsch N, Grahovac M, *et al.* Glioma survival prediction with combined analysis of *In Vivo* ^{11}C-MET pet features, *Ex Vivo* features, and patient features by supervised machine learning. J Nucl Med 2018; 59(6): 892-9.
[http://dx.doi.org/10.2967/jnumed.117.202267] [PMID: 29175980]

[51] Karhade AV, Thio Q, Ogink P, *et al.* Development of machine learning algorithms for prediction of 5-year spinal chordoma survival. World Neurosurg 2018; 119: e842-7.
[http://dx.doi.org/10.1016/j.wneu.2018.07.276] [PMID: 30096498]

[52] Janssen SJ, van der Heijden AS, van Dijke M, *et al.* Marshall urist young investigator award: prognostication in patients with long bone metastases: does a boosting algorithm improve survival estimates? Clin Orthop Relat Res 2015; 473(10): 3112-21.
[http://dx.doi.org/10.1007/s11999-015-4446-z] [PMID: 26155769]

[53] Lu C, Lewis JS Jr, Dupont WD, Plummer WD Jr, Janowczyk A, Madabhushi A. An oral cavity squamous cell carcinoma quantitative histomorphometric-based image classifier of nuclear morphology can risk stratify patients for disease-specific survival. Mod Pathol 2017; 30(12): 1655-65.
[http://dx.doi.org/10.1038/modpathol.2017.98] [PMID: 28776575]

[54] Haenssle HA, Fink C, Schneiderbauer R, *et al.* Man against machine: diagnostic performance of a deep learning convolutional neural network for dermoscopic melanoma recognition in comparison to 58 dermatologists. Ann Oncol 2018; 29(8): 1836-42.
[http://dx.doi.org/10.1093/annonc/mdy166] [PMID: 29846502]

[55] Li X, Zhang S, Zhang Q, *et al.* Diagnosis of thyroid cancer using deep convolutional neural network models applied to sonographic images: a retrospective, multicohort, diagnostic study. Lancet Oncol 2019; 20(2): 193-201.
[http://dx.doi.org/10.1016/S1470-2045(18)30762-9] [PMID: 30583848]

[56] Esteva A, Kuprel B, Novoa RA, *et al.* Dermatologist-level classification of skin cancer with deep neural networks. Nature 2017; 542(7639): 115-8.
[http://dx.doi.org/10.1038/nature21056] [PMID: 28117445]

[57] Coudray N, Ocampo PS, Sakellaropoulos T, *et al.* Classification and mutation prediction from non-small cell lung cancer histopathology images using deep learning. Nat Med 2018; 24(10): 1559-67.
[http://dx.doi.org/10.1038/s41591-018-0177-5] [PMID: 30224757]

[58] Huang S, Yang J, Fong S, Zhao Q. Artificial intelligence in cancer diagnosis and prognosis: Opportunities and challenges. Cancer Lett 2020; 471: 61-71.
[http //dx.doi.org/10.1016/j.canlet.2019.12.007] [PMID: 31830558]

[59] Leoncini L, Cossu A, Megha T, *et al.* Expression of p34(cdc2) and cyclins A and B compared to other proliferative features of non-Hodgkin's lymphomas: a multivariate cluster analysis. Int J Cancer 1999; 83(2): 203-9.

[http://dx.doi.org/10.1002/(SICI)1097-0215(19991008)83:2<203::AID-IJC10>3.0.CO;2-0]   [PMID: 10471528]

[60]   Brancati N, De Pietro G, Frucci M, Riccio D. A deep learning approach for breast invasive ductal carcinoma detection and lymphoma multi-classification in histological images. IEEE Access 2019; 7: 44709-20.
[http://dx.doi.org/10.1109/ACCESS.2019.2908724]

[61]   Tabibu S, Vinod PK, Jawahar CV. A deep learning approach for Pan-Renal Cell Carcinoma classification and survival prediction from histopathology images. bioRxiv 2019.

[62]   Haenssle HA, Fink C, Schneiderbauer R, *et al.* Man against machine: diagnostic performance of a deep learning convolutional neural network for dermoscopic melanoma recognition in comparison to 58 dermatologists. Ann Oncol 2018; 29(8): 1836-42.
[http://dx.doi.org/10.1093/annonc/mdy166] [PMID: 29846502]

CHAPTER 6

Artificial Intelligence Played an Active Role in the COVID-19 Epidemic in China

Shigao Huang[1,*], Jie Yang[2,3,4], Xianxian Liu[2], Simon Fong[2,4] and Qi Zhao[1]

[1] *Institute of Translational Medicine, Faculty of Health Sciences, University of Macau 999078, Macau SAR, China*

[2] *Department of Computer and Information Science, University of Macau, Macau, China*

[3] *Chongqing Industry & Trade Polytechnic, Chongqing, China*

[4] *Zhuhai Institutes of Advanced Technology of the Chinese Academy of Sciences, Zhuhai, China*

Abstract: This perspective aims to summarize the COVID-19 experience of the Chinese people, which included psychological assistance and open datasets. We hope that countries across the world can utilize the lessons learned and tools developed by China in response to the COVID-19 pandemic and share their fighting experience in academic publication freely so the world can solve this crisis. This perspective focuses on psychological assistance and open datasets in China's COVID-19 pandemic; they played an important role in fighting with COVID-19 and acquired major contributions to calm people in the restless environment. We hope other countries can absorb the quintessence from this experience and utilize their situation to prevent and protect citizens from being infected and get rid of sequela in the COVID-19 epidemic.

Keywords: COVID-19, Epidemic, Open datasets, Psychological assistance.

The COVID-19 pandemic, which began in Wuhan, China, has rapidly spread across the world, leading to a great loss of lives and enormous societal impacts. Wuhan-a city of China has been placed under a 76-day lockdown with strong containment measures. With restrictions scheduled to be lifted in April, residents, patients, and medical workers are all likely to be dealing with various levels of psychological trauma [1]. Psychological trauma manifests in three aspects: thinking, emotion and behavior. This novel Coronavirus is a new unknown virus having high infectious risk and lack any specific treatment. Healthcare staff has also suffered from it, and a lot of deaths have been reported.

[*] **Corresponding author Shigao Huang:** Institute of Translational Medicine, Faculty of Health Sciences, University of Macau 999078, Macau SAR, China; Tel: 853 88222953, Fax: 853 88222953; E-mail: huangshigao2010@aliyun.com

The associated fear with the pandemic can affect the victims' psychological tolerance by resulting in a series of psychological chain reactions on emotion, cognition, and behavior. COVID-19 diagnosed patients can manifest with amplified anxiety options. Additional stressors in a strictly enclosed environment like an isolation ward include unfamiliarity with medical staff and biohazard precautions, health monitoring sounds, and even seeing fellow patients dealing with the disease [2].

We hope the COVID-19 patients not only start receiving psychological assistance from medical staff but are also encouraged to engage in psychological self-help techniques such as accepting their own emotions, expressing feelings and needs, and determine specific goals to ensure a quicker recovery. Mental health has been linked to longer hospitalizations and worse outcomes in acute and chronic diseases. The mental health of the COVID-19 patient will have an impact on the length of stay and cure rate. In addition to patients, the medical staff is also susceptible to the psychological stress of this disease. With frequent contact with confirmed and suspected COVID-19 patients, health care workers may worry about the risk of contracting this highly contagious disease. Further adding to this stress is the concern of passing on the disease to loved ones at home [3]. We hope everyone can understand and support the health care workers so we may defeat our common enemy, the novel coronavirus.

In China, an evolutionary prediction system for infectious disease prevention has been established and is based on artificial intelligence (AI) methods. Steps to prevent COVID-19 disease include tracking the propagation path, screening high-risk groups, deducing the development of the epidemic situation, and providing macro decision prediction. To date, AI has been widely used in COVID-19 research. In this breaking epidemic, we also applied AI methods to improve the accuracy of COVID-19 diagnosis. Other scientists have also applied AI methods to fight the COVID-19 pandemic. We hope the research community will continue to explore and apply AI applications for COVID-19 prediction and prevention [4].

As the epidemic situation continues to change, clinical and epidemiological information is continuously released, updated, and iterated. Many data scientists and Professionals are using these data sets to efficiently sort and mine relevant patterns (such as virus hosts, mutation branches, and transmission routes) [5]. Key goals in much of this work are to quickly grasp the source of the virus outbreaks and effectively improve the clinical treatment. As of now, many Chinese Open Knowledge Graph (http://openkg.cn) datasets have been released regarding COVID-19 Pneumonia and include clinical, epidemiological prevention and control, and materials for more than 12 open knowledge graphs in other fields. Some of these include a COVID-19 health graph constructed by Tsinghua

University and Miao Health, a graph of viral drugs and virus affinities jointly constructed by Zhejiang University and Huawei Cloud, a graph of COVID-19 hotspot events constructed by Hohai University, and Wuhan University of Science and Technology [6]. Epidemiological graphs constructed by COVID-19 Materials, IBM China Research Institute, *etc*.; meanwhile, the encyclopedias from Tongji University, Zhejiang University, Southeast University, Haizhizhi Information Technology, Wen Yin Internet, Xiaomi AI Lab, Fudan University, *etc*. have been updated. It also includes Atlas, scientific research graph, clinical graph, hero graph, and other parts of the data, the COVID-19 prevention, and control graph. By using the COVID-19 scientific research graph data (http://openkg.cn/dataset/covid-19-research), data can be obtained, including the mutation pattern of the virus strain: The mining result contains the mutation branch of the COVID-19 virus, resulting in City, virus vector, and other related information are sorted by the number of occurrences. The excavation pattern revealed the details of the cities and variant branches of the 2019-nCOV strains: The source cities of the COVID-19 strains are Wuhan (21 strains), Shenzhen (8 strains), Paris (4 strains), and Hangzhou (4 Strains), Sydney (3 strains) and so on. Different cities have different mutation strains. For example, some strains in Wuhan mutate in branch 036, and some strains in Paris mutate in branch 043. These analysis results can help experts quickly understand the characteristics of COVID-19 virus strains in different cities to quickly detect the strain types and assist in the treatment [7]. The graph data in the COVID-19 graph mining system comes from the Chinese Open Knowledge Graph COVID-19 group, which is based on a unified naming convention and semantic format, and uses CC-by SA (https://creativecommons.org/) similar signature open license agreement. We also hope the global research community can benefit from this open dataset and protect the health of the public [8]. We, as the Authors, hope that countries across the world can utilize the lessons learned and tools developed in China's response to the COVID-19 pandemic and share their fighting experience in academic publication freely so the world can solve this crisis.

CONSENT FOR PUBLICATION

Not Applicable.

CONFLICT OF INTEREST

The author confirms that this chapter contents have no conflict of interest.

ACKNOWLEDGEMENT

Declared none.

REFERENCES

[1]   World Health Organization (WHO). Novel Coronavirus (2019-nCoV) situation reports. 2020.

[2]   Moorthy V, Henao Restrepo AM, Preziosi MP, Swaminathan S. Data sharing for novel coronavirus (COVID-19). Bull World Health Organ 2020; 98(3): 150.
[http://dx.doi.org/10.2471/BLT.20.251561] [PMID: 32132744]

[3]   People's Government of Hubei Province. 2020.http://www.hubei.gov.cn/zhuanti/2020/gzxxgzbd/zxtb/202003/t20200324_2189256.shtml

[4]   Huang S, Yang J, Fong S, Zhao Q. Artificial intelligence in cancer diagnosis and prognosis: Opportunities and challenges. Cancer Lett 2020; 471: 61-71.
[http://dx.doi.org/10.1016/j.canlet.2019.12.007] [PMID: 31830558]

[5]   Huang S, Yang J, Fong S, Zhao Q. Mining prognosis index of brain metastases using artificial intelligence. Cancers (Basel) 2019; 11(8): 1140.
[http://dx.doi.org/10.3390/cancers11081140] [PMID: 31395825]

[6]   Peng M, Yang J, Shi Q, *et al.* Artificial Intelligence Application in COVID-19 Diagnosis and Prediction 2020. https://ssrn.com/abstract=3541119
[http://dx.doi.org/10.2139/ssrn.3541119]

[7]   Li L, *et al.* Artificial intelligence distinguishes COVID-19 from community-acquired pneumonia on chest CT. Radiology 2020; 200905.
[http://dx.doi.org/10.1148/radiol.2020200905]

[8]   McCall B. COVID-19 and artificial intelligence: protecting health-care workers and curbing the spread. Lancet Digit Health 2020; 2(4): e166-7.
[http://dx.doi.org/10.1016/S2589-7500(20)30054-6]

CHAPTER 7

Current Status and Future Outlook of Deep Learning Techniques For Nodule Detection

Shigao Huang[1,*], Jie Yang[2,3,4], Kun Lan[2], Sunny Yaoyang Wu[2], Simon Fong[2,4] and Qi Zhao[1]

[1] *Institute of Translational Medicine, Faculty of Health Sciences, University of Macau, Macau SAR, China*

[2] *Department of Computer and Information Science, University of Macau, Macau, China*

[3] *Chongqing Industry & Trade Polytechnic, Chongqing, China*

[4] *Zhuhai Institutes of Advanced Technology of the Chinese Academy of Sciences, Zhuhai, China*

Abstract: This chapter reports that Artificial Intelligence (AI) in clinical oncology includes deep learning for detecting the lung nodules and other algorithms for analyzing the nodules to acquire an early diagnosis of nodules and tumors. Therefore, the early diagnosis is of great significance in the treatment of lung cancer or pre-cancerous disease. Also, the early detection of nodules can improve the treatment effects and reduce the chance of misdiagnosis.

Keywords: Artificial intelligence, Deep learning, Lung nodule, Lung nodule detection, Nodule detection.

1. INTRODUCTION

Lung cancer is a common malignant tumor that poses a great threat to life and health. Currently, the incidence and mortality rate of lung cancer is very high [1]. Among all malignant neoplasms, lung cancer has the second-highest incidence, mortality, and morbidity among women and men. The cause of lung cancer is not completely clear. Numerous research data have shown that high doses of smoking are closely related to the development of lung cancer [2]. At present, the most effective way to prolong the survival time of lung cancer patients is early diagnosis. Therefore, early diagnosis and treatment of lung cancer and pre-cancerous diseases are of great importance.

* **Corresponding author Shigao Huang:** Institute of Translational Medicine, Faculty of Health Sciences, University of Macau 999078, Macau SAR, China; Tel: 853 88222953, Fax: 853 88222953; E-mail: huangshigao2010@aliyun.com

Pulmonary Nodules (PNs) are usually seen on high-resolution CT [3]. PN can be single or multiple in the lung and appear dense, ≤3 cm in diameter, rounded or slightly irregular in shape, with clear or blurred borders on imaging. In the clinical presentation, there are usually no obvious symptoms and signs, and it is often diagnosed in the health check-up. In recent years, with the improvement of living standards and the awareness of national health check-ups, more lung nodules have been detected [4]. As a result, pulmonary nodules have gradually become a hot issue discussed by researchers here at home and abroad. The causes of pulmonary nodules are still unclear, and many lung diseases may result in the formation of lung nodules. Fig **(1)** shows the framework of AI distinguished computerized tomography and various kinds of objects to be targeted. In a statistical analysis of a large population, it was found that more than half of the small nodules with a single diameter of >25px were malignant [4, 5]. This data suggest that nodules that are often discovered unintentionally during the physical examination should not be taken lightly.

Therefore, it is particularly important to improve the detection rate and diagnostic accuracy of pulmonary nodules. The rapid development of computer science has brought Artificial Intelligence (AI) into the limelight and has been gradually applied in medical research [5, 6]. In particular, Deep Learning (DL) technology is more widely being used in imaging research. This paper reviews the current status of AI and DL techniques in PN detection.

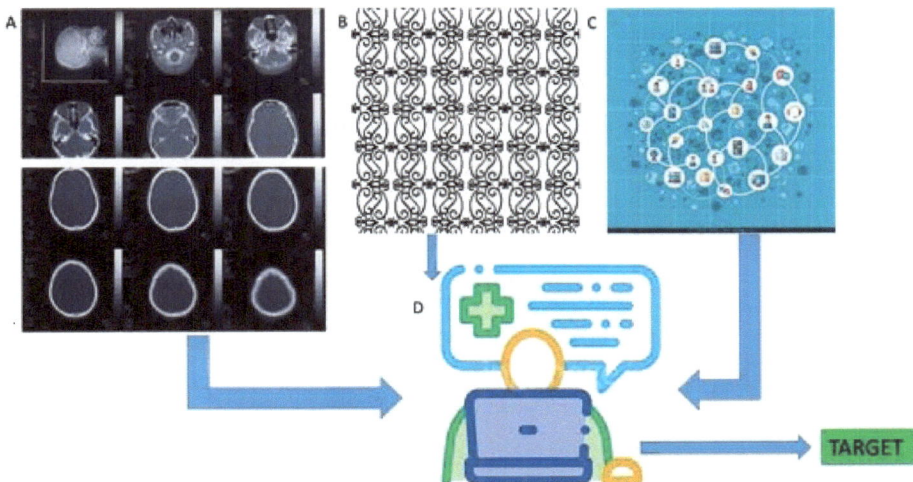

Fig. (1). The framework of AI distinguished computerized tomography (CT) imaging **(A)**, various shapes **(B)**, and Social activity **(C)** from the number of objectives to acquire the target. A: some nodules in CT image to be verified by AI.

2. OVERVIEW OF PULMONARY NODULES

Pulmonary nodules are defined as rounded or oval-shaped growth in the lungs that appear as irregular opacity, measuring ≤3 cm in diameter in focal high-density images of the lung [7]. It can be solid or subsolid and can be solitary or multiple. These are usually not associated with pulmonary insufficiency, pleural effusion, and portal lymph node swelling [8]. There are several ways to classify PN, according to size; <5mm for microscopic nodules and 5-10mm for small nodules [9].

Nodules, according to density, can be divided into two categories of solid and subsolid; the latter is divided into Ground Glass Nodule (GGN) and partially solid nodules [10]. Pulmonary nodules usually have no obvious signs and symptoms and are usually found during a health check-up [11]. Pulmonary pathogenesis of nodules is not fully understood, and many diseases of the lung can trigger the development of these nodules, so the possible diagnoses of pulmonary nodules may be tuberculosis balls, malignant tumors, fungal infections, inflammatory pseudotumors, sclerosing lung cell tumors [12], and as well as other benign or malignant metastases and primary lung cancers. The most common cause of solitary malignant nodule is primary lung cancer, accounting for approximately 75% of cases [13]. Multiple malignant nodules are most frequently the result of metastatic tumors, including lymphoma, smooth muscle sarcoma, and malignant teratoma, *etc.* Some of the benign lesions may also turn malignant with time. Methods of assessing pulmonary nodules generally include tumor markers, imaging, functional imaging, surgical and non-surgical biopsies. Any clinical information, such as the patient's history of smoking, history of cancer, sex, age, occupation, history of chronic lung disease, treatment of relevant diseases, and referral, can also be of great help in assessing PN.

3. OVERVIEW OF AI AND DEEP LEARNING

A group of scientists, led by McCarthy, Rochester, Minsky, and Shenon, gathered at Dartmouth College in the summer of 1956 [14] to explore questions about the use of machines to simulate intelligence and, for the first time, to propose an "artificial intelligence" [15]. AI is part of computer science, which is a new discipline. It is a new science and technology that may be described as a theory, method, technique, or primarily applied system.

It is used to simulate and extend human intelligence. AI is dedicated to understand the essence of intelligence and generate intelligence that can do the same thing as humans do since Intelligent machines respond similarly. One of its examples can be seen when expert systems, robotics, natural language processing, and language image recognition are utilized in a chess match [15]. Furthermore, Grandmaster Kasparov was also invited by IBM [16] to participate in the Deep Blue research project [17], and in the end, an IBM supercomputer defeated the world chess champion Kasparov in a chess match. Fig. (2) shows the multiple developments of AI applications in the surgery process and other fields such as the robot, human-robot, neuroscience, language talking, *etc.* These are undoubtedly the perfect examples of AI [18]. AI can think like the human mind. But it is not the same as human intelligence [19], it is a kind of information process that simulates human consciousness and thinking, and it is very likely to surpass humans. In recent years, the theory and technology of AI have become increasingly mature and widely used in a variety of different fields [20].

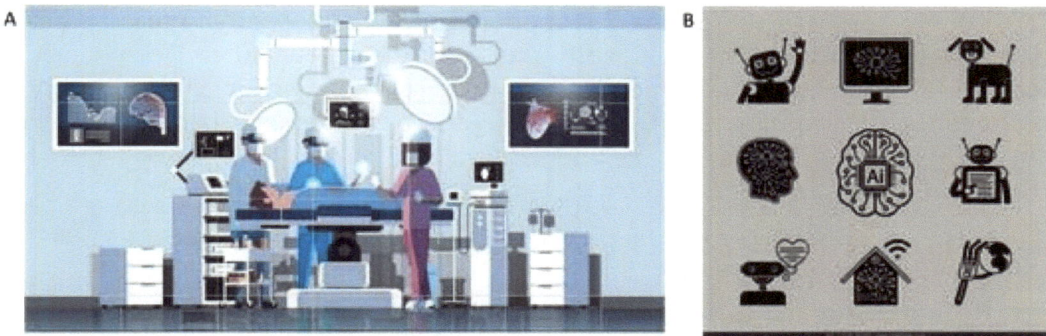

Fig. (2). AI application in surgery process **(A)** and AI application in multiple activities **(B)**. A: machine learning *vs.* traditional methods in the surgery process, utilize computer algorithm to find the surgery window to perform, then execute location. B: AI application in robot dog, human-robot, neuroscience, language talking, *et al.*

In 2006, Geoffrey Hinton *et al.* first proposed the concept of "deep learning" in Science, a leading academic journal, marking the formal birth of deep learning technology research. The introduction of DL brings machine learning closer to the original goal of "artificial intelligence" [21]. Deep learning has a range of learning algorithms such as Convolutional Neural Networks (CNN) [22], Autoencoder (AE) [23], and Recurrent Neural Network (RNN) [24].

In recent years, with the development in deep learning technology, it has also been widely used in medical research [25 - 29], especially in the shadowing idea of Liu *et al.* [30]. Moreover, CNN is also used to classify PET and brain magnetic resonance images. A bimodal imaging data evaluation framework based on deep learning is proposed and applied in Alzheimer's disease. This framework was found to yield higher classification accuracy. The DL technique was used to study the results, which showed that the diagnosis of pneumothorax, pulmonary edema, pleural effusion, and solid lung lesions were all highly effective.

The true positive rates were 78%, 82%, 91%, and 74%, respectively. Shickel *et al.* [31] put patients with schizophrenia and healthy controls in a static state. The image data collected by the information state fMRI were classified using a deep neural network model (DNN), and the results showed that the ability of CNN models could also be utilized in studies of preterm infants. Furthermore, Kawahara *et al.* used an improved CNN model that was able to predict the neurodevelopmental status of the preterm brain network and skin diseases.

In a study, Esteva *et al.* [32] created a skin cancer diagnostic system based on a CNN model with high accuracy of 69.4%, which is equivalent to 66.0% of a dermatologist's diagnostic level. In colonography, Suzuki *et al.* used the DL algorithm to automatically detect colonic polyps. In studies related to the breast [33], Wang *et al.* [34] used the CNN model in breast occupancy to make a better distinction between cystic and soft tissue density occupancy. Deep learning technology has been applied and achieved good results in breast cancer detection, malignancy determination, differential diagnosis, and other aspects of relevant studies.

4. APPLICATION OF DEEP LEARNING IN LUNG NODULES

4.1. Rationale for the Detection of Pulmonary Nodules

The main principle is the recognition of images in deep learning techniques to detect nodules. It includes four processes: collecting data, pre-processing the image, segmenting the image, and detecting the nodules. Among them, the detection of nodules is the core of current research. Detection methods generally include a threshold-based method [35], template matching method, shape enhancement filter method, clustering method, and so on. Regardless of the method, a high false-positive rate is a great challenge. To screen out false-positive nodules, the classification of nodules is mostly processed using support vector machines, artificial neural networks, linear discriminant analysis, and other methods.

4.2. Application of Deep Learning in the Detection and Diagnosis of Pulmonary Nodules

In recent years, the DL algorithm has been used extensively to detect pulmonary nodules and has been shown to have good sensitivity. Computer-aided Detection [36] and Diagnosis (CAD) in conventional pulmonary nodules are being widely used [37]. The system applies a multi-view CNN model that shows its performance in a much better way than traditional CAD. The true-positive rate of characterization can be as high as 85%. Low-dose thin-layer CT scans are being widely used in China at present.

It fully meets the technical requirements for DL detection of pulmonary nodules. For example, Mohammad *et al.* [38] used CAD to detect a 1mm CT image, and the true positive rate of detection was as high as 98% for lung nodules >3mm in diameter [38]. In the study of tube current correlation, Hein *et al.* found that a decrease in the tube current did not cause a difference in the detection of pulmonary nodules. In a tubular voltage study, Yaxley *et al.* [38, 39] found that differences in tubular voltage did not cause significant differences in test results.

The diagnostic imaging of PN is the result of a diagnostic radiologist's assessment of the benign and malignant nature of the nodal lesions on X-ray and CT images. An accurate judgment can provide good direction for clinical treatment, and computer-aided diagnostic systems can greatly assist the physicians due to their ability to quickly identify lesions and assess their benign or malignant nature, thereby greatly improving the quality of healthcare. Using a CNN classification model with multiscale inputs, Ying *et al.* found that the three types of CNNs could be classified into three different categories [40].

Images of pulmonary nodules at different scales are inputs that allow a more accurate and comprehensive assessment of nodule characteristics and then feature the data. Kim *et al.* [41] applied a method to identify pulmonary nodules and obtained an accuracy of 95.5%. It was also found that with the help of an AI computer-aided diagnostic system, the diagnostic accuracy of the physicians was significantly improved. Another study on 1012 pulmonary nodules in the LIDC-IDRI database resulted in a significant increase in the accuracy of the diagnosis. The area under the ROC curve was 0.927 for predicting benign and malignant properties using texture characterization.

The deep learning techniques have a great ability to detect benign and malignant pulmonary nodules in the chest CT. Although deep learning techniques have been widely used and show great advantages in the diagnosis of pulmonary nodules, they have certain limitations and problems that need to be solved. At present, the main focus is on learning from tagged data. A large number of details are untagged, and manual tagging wastes a lot of time. Therefore, future research should focus on how to automate the tagging of data.

Besides, the training accuracy is directly proportional to the training time. If you go for speed, you will sacrifice part of the accuracy. However, an increased training accuracy will extend the training time. Therefore, the focus of research is now on how to ensure training accuracy and reduce training time. Besides, it is also recommended that the relevant parties should authoritatively evaluate the diagnosis of AI in pulmonary nodules, an important adjunct for physicians in making a diagnosis of pulmonary nodules. In a tubular current correlation study, Hein *et al.* found that a decrease in tubular current did not cause pulmonary nodule detection results.

Regarding the tube voltage study, Doris *et al.* found that differences in tube voltage did not cause significant [42] differences. The diagnostic imaging of PN is the process by which the diagnostic radiologist examines the benign and malignant nature of the nodal lesions on X-rays and CT images.

An accurate judgment pair can provide good direction for clinical treatment and physicians are greatly assisted by the ability of a computer-aided diagnostic system to quickly identify lesions and assess their benign or malignant nature, thereby greatly improving the quality of care. Using a CNN classification model with multiscale inputs, it was also found that the diagnostic accuracy of physicians was significantly improved with the help of an AI computer-aided diagnostic system. Another study used textural feature analysis to predict the benign and malignant nature of 1012 pulmonary nodules in the LIDC-IDRI database, with an area under the ROC curve was 0.927.

5. DATABASE

Databases can generally be divided into two main categories: One used for testing and the other used for training. There are five main databases for training: the 2017 Ali Tenchi Competition training dataset; Kaggle Data Science, Bowl2017 training dataset; LTRC-ILD database; The Nelson trial database; LIDC-IDRI database. The LTRC-ILD has 533 data sets, and the rest of the databases have more than 1000 data sets. Furthermore, there are three databases used for testing, the 2017 Ali Tenchi Competition test dataset, the Kaggle Data Science Bowl 2017 test dataset, and the ANODE09 database. They relatively process small data compared to the training databases.

6. ISSUES AND OUTLOOK

Although deep learning techniques have been widely used and shown great advantages in the diagnosis of pulmonary nodules, they still have some limitations and problems that need to be resolved. At present, the main focus is on learning from tagged data. Therefore, future research should focus on how to automate the tagging of data. Besides, the training accuracy is directly proportional to training time. If you go for speed, you will sacrifice part of the accuracy, and increasing the training accuracy will extend the training time. Therefore, the focus of research is now on how to ensure training accuracy and reduce training time. Thus making a diagnosis of pulmonary nodules by AI is an important adjunct for doctors.

CONSENT FOR PUBLICATION

Not Applicable.

CONFLICT OF INTEREST

The author confirms that this chapter contents have no conflict of interest.

ACKNOWLEDGEMENT

Declared none.

REFERENCES

[1]   Pless M, Stupp R, Ris HB, *et al.* Induction chemoradiation in stage IIIA/N2 non-small-cell lung cancer: a phase 3 randomised trial. Lancet 2015; 386(9998): 1049-56.
        [http://dx.doi.org/10.1016/S0140-6736(15)60294-X] [PMID: 26275735]

[2]   Torre LA, Siegel RL, Jemal A. Lung cancer statistics.Lung cancer and personalized medicine. Springer 2016; pp. 1-19.
        [http://dx.doi.org/10.1007/978-3-319-24223-1_1]

[3]   Mori S, Cho I, Koga Y, Sugimoto M. Comparison of pulmonary abnormalities on high-resolution computed tomography in patients with early *versus* longstanding rheumatoid arthritis. J Rheumatol 2008; 35(8): 1513-21.
        [PMID: 18597412]

[4]   MacMahon H, Naidich DP, Goo JM, *et al.* Guidelines for management of incidental pulmonary nodules detected on CT images: from the Fleischner Society 2017. Radiology 2017; 284(1): 228-43.
        [http://dx.doi.org/10.1148/radiol.2017161659] [PMID: 28240562]

[5]   Naidich DP, Bankier AA, MacMahon H, *et al.* Recommendations for the management of subsolid pulmonary nodules detected at CT: a statement from the Fleischner Society. Radiology 2013; 266(1): 304-17.
        [http://dx.doi.org/10.1148/radiol.12120628] [PMID: 23070270]

[6]   Khan A, *et al.* A survey of the recent architectures of deep convolutional neural networks. Artif Intell Rev 2020; 1-62.

[7]   Nemanic S, London CA, Wisner ER. Comparison of thoracic radiographs and single breath-hold helical CT for detection of pulmonary nodules in dogs with metastatic neoplasia. J Vet Intern Med 2006; 20(3): 508-15.
        [http://dx.doi.org/10.1111/j.1939-1676.2006.tb02889.x] [PMID: 16734082]

[8]   Khan AN, Al-Jahdali HH, Allen CM, Irion KL, Al Ghanem S, Koteyar SS. The calcified lung nodule: What does it mean? Ann Thorac Med 2010; 5(2): 67-79.
        [http://dx.doi.org/10.4103/1817-1737.62469] [PMID: 20582171]

[9]   Edey AJ, Hansell DM. Incidentally detected small pulmonary nodules on CT. Clin Radiol 2009; 64(9): 872-84.
        [http://dx.doi.org/10.1016/j.crad.2009.03.006] [PMID: 19664477]

[10]   Travis WD, *et al.* The IASLC lung cancer staging project: proposals for coding T categories for

sub-solid nodules and assessment of tumor size in part-solid tumors in the forthcoming eighth edition of the TNM classification of lung cancer. J Thoracic Oncol 2016; 11(8): 1204-23.

[11] Odry BL, *et al.* Solid component evaluation in mixed ground-glass nodules. Medical Imaging 2007: Image Processing. International Society for Optics and Photonics 2007.
[http://dx.doi.org/10.1117/12.709892]

[12] Patel VK, Naik SK, Naidich DP, *et al.* A practical algorithmic approach to the diagnosis and management of solitary pulmonary nodules: part 1: radiologic characteristics and imaging modalities. Chest 2013; 143(3): 825-39.
[http://dx.doi.org/10.1378/chest.12-0960] [PMID: 23460160]

[13] Evangelista L, *et al.* Ground glass pulmonary nodules: their significance in oncology patients and the role of computer tomography and 18F–fluorodeoxyglucose positron emission tomography. European J Hybrid Imaging 2018; 2(1): 2.

[14] Rose F. Into the heart of the mind: an American quest for artificial intelligence. Frank Rose 1985.

[15] Ekmekci PE, Arda B. Artificial Intelligence and Bioethics. Springer 2020.
[http://dx.doi.org/10.1007/978-3-030-52448-7]

[16] Hsu F-h. IBM's deep blue chess grandmaster chips. IEEE Micro 1999; 19(2): 70-81.
[http://dx.doi.org/10.1109/40.755469]

[17] Durkin J. 4 Expert System. The Handbook of Applied Expert Systems 1997; 4: 15.

[18] Biri SA. Artificial intelligence, machine learning, deep learning, and cognitive computing: what do these terms mean and how will they impact health care? J Arthroplasty 2018; 33(8): 2358-61.
[http://dx.doi.org/10.1016/j.arth.2018.02.067] [PMID: 29656964]

[19] Copeland J. Artificial intelligence: A philosophical introduction. John Wiley & Sons 2015.

[20] Pachet F. Computer analysis of jazz chord sequence: is solar a blues? 2000.

[21] Hinton G, *et al.* Deep neural networks for acoustic modeling in speech recognition: The shared views of four research groups. IEEE Signal Process Mag 2012; 29(6): 82-97.
[http://dx.doi.org/10.1109/MSP.2012.2205597]

[22] Shin W, Bu S-J, Cho S-B. 3D-convolutional neural network with generative adversarial network and autoencoder for robust anomaly detection in video surveillance. Int J Neural Syst 2020; 30(6)2050034
[http://dx.doi.org/10.1142/S0129065720500343] [PMID: 32466693]

[23] Kiran BR, Thomas DM, Parakkal R. An overview of deep learning-based methods for unsupervised and semi-supervised anomaly detection in videos. J Imaging 2018; 4(2): 36.
[http://dx.doi.org/10.3390/jimaging4020036]

[24] Gensler A, *et al.* Deep Learning for solar power forecasting—An approach using AutoEncoder and LSTM Neural Networks in 2016 IEEE international conference on systems, man, and cybernetics (SMC). IEEE 2016.

[25] Kuramoto T, *et al.* Time series forecasting using a deep belief network with restricted Boltzmann machines. Neurocomputing 2014; 137: 47-56.
[http://dx.doi.org/10.1016/j.neucom.2013.03.047]

[26] Zhang H, *et al.* Stackgan: Text to photo-realistic image synthesis with stacked generative adversarial networks. Proceedings of the IEEE international conference on computer vision.
[http://dx.doi.org/10.1109/ICCV.2017.629]

[27] Alom MZ, *et al.* 2018.

[28] Alom MZ, *et al.* A state-of-the-art survey on deep learning theory and architectures. Electronics (Basel) 2019; 8(3): 292.
[http://dx.doi.org/10.3390/electronics8030292]

[29] Lee J-G, Jun S, Cho YW, *et al.* Deep learning in medical imaging: general overview. Korean J Radiol

2017; 18(4): 570-84.
[http://dx.doi.org/10.3348/kjr.2017.18.4.570] [PMID: 28670152]

[30]   Liu S, *et al.* Deep learning in medical ultrasound analysis: a review. Engineering 2019; 5(2): 261-75.
[http://dx.doi.org/10.1016/j.eng.2018.11.020]

[31]   Shickel B, Tighe PJ, Bihorac A, Rashidi P. Deep EHR: a survey of recent advances in deep learning techniques for electronic health record (EHR) analysis. IEEE J Biomed Health Inform 2018; 22(5): 1589-604.
[http://dx.doi.org/10.1109/JBHI.2017.2767063] [PMID: 29989977]

[32]   Esteva A, *et al.* Dermatologist-level classification of skin cancer with deep neural networks. Nature 2017; 542(7639): 115-8.

[33]   Xu J, *et al.* Massive-training support vector regression with feature selection in application of computer-aided detection of polyps in ct colonography.Emerging Developments and Practices in Oncology. IGI Global 2018; pp. 153-90.
[http://dx.doi.org/10.4018/978-1-5225-3085-5.ch006]

[34]   Wang Y, Wang N, Xu M, *et al.* Deeply-supervised networks with threshold loss for cancer detection in automated breast ultrasound. IEEE Trans Med Imaging 2020; 39(4): 866-76.
[http://dx.doi.org/10.1109/TMI.2019.2936500] [PMID: 31442972]

[35]   Gros C. Automatic Segmentation of Intramedullary Multiple Sclerosis Lesions. École Polytechnique de Montréal 2018.

[36]   Shin H-C, Roth HR, Gao M, *et al.* Deep convolutional neural networks for computer-aided detection: CNN architectures, dataset characteristics, and transfer learning. IEEE Trans Med Imaging 2016; 35(5): 1285-98.
[http://dx.doi.org/10.1109/TMI.2016.2528162] [PMID: 26886976]

[37]   Hua K-L, Hsu CH, Hidayati SC, Cheng WH, Chen YJ. Computer-aided classification of lung nodules on computed tomography images *via* deep learning technique. OncoTargets Ther 2015; 8: 2015-22.
[PMID: 26346558]

[38]   Al Mohammad B, Brennan PC, Mello-Thoms C. A review of lung cancer screening and the role of computer-aided detection. Clin Radiol 2017; 72(6): 433-42.
[http://dx.doi.org/10.1016/j.crad.2017.01.002] [PMID: 28185635]

[39]   Yaxley J, Pirrone C. Review of the diagnostic evaluation of renal tubular acidosis. Ochsner J 2016; 16(4): 525-30.
[PMID: 27999512]

[40]   Li Y, *et al.* Deep learning for remote sensing image classification: A survey. WIREs Data Mining and Knowledge Discovery 2018; 8(6)e1264
[http://dx.doi.org/10.1002/widm.1264]

[41]   Kim B-C, Sung YS, Suk H-I. Deep feature learning for pulmonary nodule classification in a lung CT. 4th International Winter Conference on Brain-Computer Interface (BCI).. IEEE 2016.

[42]   Leithner D, Wichmann JL, Mahmoudi S, *et al.* Diagnostic yield of 90-kVp low-tube-voltage carotid and intracerebral CT-angiography: effects on radiation dose, image quality and diagnostic performance for the detection of carotid stenosis. Br J Radiol 2018; 91(1086): 20170927-.
[http://dx.doi.org/10.1259/bjr.20170927] [PMID: 29493282]

CHAPTER 8

Artificial Intelligence-Based Mining of Benign and Malignant Characteristics of Pulmonary Ground-Glass Nodules

Xiaoxia Li[1], Ting Gao[2] and Shigao Huang[3,*]

[1] *Shaanxi ZeEr HuiEr Education Technology Co. LTD, Shaanxi, Xi'an, China*

[2] *Baoji Vocational and Technical College, Baoji, Shaan Xi, China*

[3] *Institute of Translational Medicine, Faculty of Health Sciences, University of Macau, Macau SAR, China*

Abstract: Deep learning-based Artificial Intelligence (AI) with medical imaging cooperation has led to a significant increase in the detection rate of early lung cancer, but the identification of its benign and malignant nature remains difficult. This chapter describes the effect of AI on CT values, maximum surface area, volume, 3D longitudinal diameter, solid occupancy, multiplication time, and also ground glass pulmonary nodule. We believe that AI will be able to provide a variety of features for the analysis of the characteristics of the world's largest and most complex computer systems. It helps radiologists to determine the benign and malignant nature of pulmonary ground-glass nodules and improves the accuracy and quality of diagnosis. Besides, patient's survival rate and quality of life can be improved as well.

Keywords: Artificial intelligence, Deep learning, Malignant characteristics, Pulmonary ground-glass nodules, Quality of life.

In recent years, with big data and Artificial Intelligence (AI) based on deep learning and the rapid rise of advanced technologies, AI has been utilized rapidly in all fields, especially in the medical field for pulmonary nodules. The application of section detection can help physicians to quickly detect pulmonary nodules and predict their benign and malignant nature at an early stage. Lung cancer screening, diagnosis, and treatment play an important role in the detection of pulmonary nodules by AI technology. AI technology has roughly experienced the development process of the image processing method, the classical machine learning method, the deep learning method, *etc* [1]. It has the advantages of learn-

* **Corresponding author Shigao Huang:** Institute of Translational Medicine, Faculty of Health Sciences, University of Macau 999078, Macau SAR, China; Tel: 853 88222953; Fax: 853 88222953; E-mail: huangshigao2010@aliyun.com

ability, universality, and high efficiency [2]. AI-based on deep learning is used to treat lung diseases. The research progress of CT characteristic quantitative parameters of the vitreous nodule is also reviewed [3].

1. DESCRIPTION OF AI

Geoffrey Hinton *et al.* first proposed the concept of Deep Learning (DL) in 2006 [4]. Deep learning belongs to an important branch of machine learning, which is AI. As a subset of Artificial Intelligence (AI), deep learning adopts the professional technique of artificial neural network algorithm. Therefore, experts believe that deep learning and artificial neural network terms are interchangeable. Deep learning in recent years, in the field of AI, is the method to mainly simulate the thinking and algorithm of the human brain, such as learning, reasoning, images, sound, *etc.* The advantage of deep learning over traditional machine learning is that it is good at processing images, voice and text. Features are not extracted manually but automatically, so we feed the system raw data images directly, and an ideal result can be achieved in a learning network. Furthermore, a deep learning algorithm is the most powerful algorithm [5]. Due to its great potential and strong processing ability, it can adapt to a variety of data. And by using simple algorithms, it can be extended to large data sets. There are many models of deep learning, and the convolutional neural network in the discriminative depth structure is among one of them [6]. The name CNNs "convolutional neural network" indicates that the network employs a mathematical operation called convolution. Convolutional networks are a specialized type of neural network that uses convolution in place of general matrix multiplication in at least one of their layers. . Deep learning is the most successful and popular network model that is widely used in medical image processing. On the other hand, the convolutional neural network has outstanding advantages in image classification and target detection. The radiology department generates hundreds of thousands or even millions of images which is a huge amount of data. The traditional computer-aided detection method has been unable to solve the problem of large data volume as they involve manual work, that is why AI is employed here. In small cases, traditional classical machine learning algorithms can be superior to deep learning [7]. On the other hand, traditional computer-aided detection methods require manual extraction of many features, the characteristics of patients and lesions are constantly changing, that is why the traditional methods are neither accurate nor durable. CNN does not need to manually design and extract features of the lung. In terms of detection of a tubercle, this network model, with the use of training data sets, automatically selects the best image. The larger the data volume, the higher the accuracy of the pulmonary tubercle characteristics obtained, and the deeper the learning. The network model is consistent with the current development situation and can be used as a long-term effective system to assist the diagnosis of pulmonary nodules.

2. DEFINITION AND CLASSIFICATION OF GROUND-GLASS NODULES

Ground-glass Nodule (GGN) is defined in imageology as local areas of lung ambiguity increased on CT images. This is manifested as a poorly defined intrapulmonary glassy opacity with normal interpulmonary density. Qualitative, pneumato-containing bronchial tubes and high-density blood vessel images [8] were used to distinguish pure ground glass (pGGN) and mixed ground glass based on solid components it contained. Ground glass nodules are pGGN if they do not contain any solid components; If it contains solid components, it is mGGN, which is also called partial solid density nodules, with a maximum diameter of ≤3cm, and pGGN and mGGN are collectively referred to as nodules or semi-nodules. For the Study of Lung Cancer (IASLC), the European Respiratory Society, ERS, and the American Thoracic Society (ATS) have released this lung adenocarcinoma. International multidisciplinary classification [9], the new classification shows molecular biology, pathology, imaging, and the latest therapies. In this new classification, lung adenocarcinoma is mainly divided into two categories: preinvasive lesions and invasive lesions, namely immersion. Prerun lesions include atypical adenomatous hyperplasia (AAH) and principal margin. Adenocarcinoma *in situ* (AIS), infiltration changes include micro-infiltration adenocarcinoma (resumes), Invasive adenocarcinoma (MIA), invasive adenocarcinoma (IAC). The new classification also emphasizes the linear progression of lung adenocarcinoma [10, 11], AAH→AIS→MIA→IAC, which are pathological tissues. Morphology is a continuous process of change. The pathological diagnosis of AIS and MIA must be obtained by surgical biopsy. The 5-year survival rate after AIS and 5-year disease-free survival rate after MIA can reach 100%.

3. ANALYSIS OF BENIGN AND MALIGNANT CHARACTERISTICS OF GROUND-GLASS NODULES

AI-based on deep learning is used for diagnosis and research in the aspect of conventional lesion characterization of ground glass nodules in the lung. Fig. (**1**) showed the difference between AI and traditional CT images. The study, such as nodule size, foliation sign and burr sign, pleural endoscopy sign, vascular bundle sign or vascular embedding sign, cavitation. Signs, *etc.*, also provide more characteristic analysis, mainly involved in the following aspects: CT value (including the largest value, minimum value, average value, kurtosis, skewness, *etc*.), maximum surface area (the 2D layer where the maximum length diameter is located area), volume, 3D diameter, compactness (a measure of the compactness of the lesion shape relative to the sphere), sphere Shape (a measure of the roundness of a lesion relative to the shape of a sphere), *etc*.

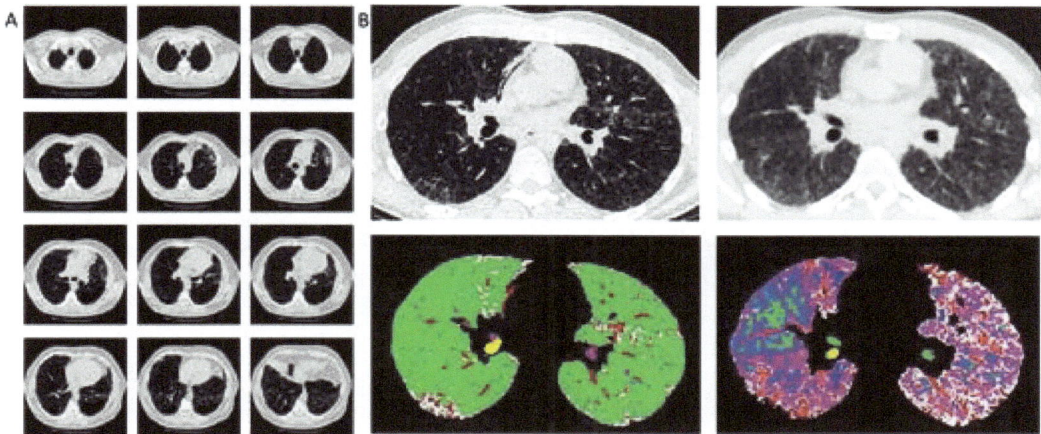

Fig. (1). Nine axial images **A)** in traditional computer tomography(CT) and the corresponding classification results (B) *via* computer aid –design (CAD) in the lung cross-section size. Note that this image is with emphysema and pulmonary fibrosis. Part of the photograph was cited from Chien, K. C. C. (2011) NNT: 2011TELE0021 [40].

3.1. CT Value

CT value is defined as a uniform unit of measurement used to represent tissue density in CT image measurement, known as Heinz. Hounsfield unit HU, which reflects changes in the lesion density for uncertain lung. The increased density of nodules indicates a greater likelihood of malignancy, which requires shorter follow-up or biopsy [12]. The ground glass nodule is often small, and the error is often larger than the traditional manual measurement method. AI with obvious advantages can quickly and accurately measure the maximum, minimum, and average CT value of lesions. Value, kurtosis, and skewness, *etc*., were studied based on the equality [11] in 97 cases of ground-glass nodules, and the maximum and average CT values were obtained. The value was statistically significant in precancerous lesions and invasive lesions, while the minimum CT value was not statistically significant in the pathological types. When the average CT value was -557HU, the sensitivity and specificity of differentiating between precancerous and invasive lesions were achieved 86.2%, 93.7%, respectively. When the mean CT value was -484HU, the sensitivity and specificity of the diagnosis of micro invasion and infiltration were determined. The heterogeneity was higher, reaching 94.4% and 96.6%. Li [13] *et al*. analyzed the realism of 207 cases (216 lesions). It was concluded that the critical values between AAH/AIS and MIA, MIA, and IAC were -548.00Hu and -364.59Hu, respectively. Li *et al.* [14] reported that when the CT value of pGGN was greater than -472HU, it was suggested to be invasive adenocarcinoma (IAC). During the follow-up of 102 ground-glass nodules, changes in CT peak values were found to help identify precancerous lesions and infiltrates Lesions [15]. The study of Horton *et al.* [16] showed the maximum, minimum, average, kurtosis, skewness, and value of CT. The percentiles were not statistically significant.

3.2. Maximum Surface Area

The maximum surface area is the area of the plane where the AI measures the maximum diameter in 2D in our lung. The nodules are shaped like irregular geometric shapes, with rounded or circular edges and irregular edges. For lobules or burrs, it is difficult for us to accurately determine the maximum section of pulmonary nodules, but AI is a good solution. To solve this problem, however, the change in the maximum surface area reflects the lesion change process to a certain extent. Ohtsuka *et al.* [17] studied a total of 163 pure ground-glass nodules which were confirmed as malignant by surgical pathology and obtained the maximum surface area as 2.224 cm^2, and the sensitivity and specificity for determining non-invasive and invasive lesions were respectively, 72.1%, 75.1%, and through logistics regression analysis showed that the maximum cross-sectional area of the pure ground-glass nodule was the diagnosis independent of invasive cancer.

Travis. *et al.* [18] also reported that the maximum surface area could help GGN differentiate from cancer. The difference between precancerous and micro-invasive lesions and infiltrating lesions was not uniform. Some studies [10, 19] showed that the maximum surface area was the most significant predictor of the growth of pulmonary nodules. However, Ma *et al.* [20] showed that there was no statistically significant difference between the maximum surface area and the invasive type of pulmonary nodules. There is a lack of uniformity in the related literature reports.

3.3. Three-Dimensional Volume

The algorithm of AI can make very accurate data on the three-dimensional volume of pulmonary nodules in related literature reports [21]. Three-dimensional volume measurement has obvious advantages over-dimensional and two - dimensional measurement in the pathologic growth pattern of the ground-glass nodule. Most of them grow in the form of accumulation or expansion, and the change of lesion volume and growth mode will become indispensable to affect patients, which enables clinicians to provide patients with more accurate treatment on time [20]. The study of 78 cases of GGN yielded volume that was helpful to distinguish invasive adenocarcinoma from precancerous or micro-invasive adenocarcinoma, and the specificity of invasive adenocarcinoma was 94.7% when ≥1.45cm was used as the threshold value. Gray *et al.* [22] conducted a total study that 163 pure ground-glass nodules were confirmed as malignant by surgery and pathology, and the threshold of the 3D volume was 1.34cm3. The sensitivity and specificity of the non-invasive and invasive lesions were 81.2% and 67.2%, respectively. Gupta. *et al.* [23] reported that the repeatable line of GGN automatic volume measurement was very good, and GGN could be confirmed when the volume increased by 27% the growth rate. Chae *et al.* [24] reported that the change of GGN volume was significantly different between precancerous lesions and invasive lesions.

3.4. Three-D Length to Diameter

With the change of lesion size, the degree of malignancy also changes. The larger the lesion, the higher the degree of malignancy. The smaller the lesion, the lower the degree of malignancies, ranging from AAH/AIS to MIA to IAC. As the size of the lesion increased gradually, the length and the diameter of the lesion could be used as an important reference to determine its benign and malignant properties. The traditional method of measurement is to select the maximum cross-section of GGN, while the 3D length and diameter are automatically measured by AI in 3D space. The data obtained by quantitative calculation is more accurate and has strong repeatability and objectivity. Yankelevitz *et al.* [25] believe that THREE-DIMENSIONAL technology has more advantages than two-dimensional technology in evaluating tumor diameter measurement, especially for nodules of irregular shape. N.P Etrick *et al.* [26] reported that radiologists and 3D tools were used to measure the lesion length. The relative deviation of diameter is -1.8%, -0.4%, -0.7%, -0.4% and -1.6%, 10mm spherical and 20mm spherical, respectively. The relative deviations of elliptic, 10mm lobulated and 10mm nodules were 1.4%, -0.1%, -26.5%, respectively 7.8% and 39.8%. The deviation of 3d measurement was significantly less than that of 1D for elliptic, lobulated, and micronodular nodules deviation. For lobulated nodules, the variation in one-dimensional measurements was significantly smaller than that for elliptic and micronodular nodules. The change has been much greater. The increase in length and the diameter of GGN was defined. As the maximum length diameter was at least 2mm greater than the original length diameter [24]. Yin *Et al* [27] reported the average diameter (OR=0.137, GGN was an independent risk factor for IAC. Lee *et al.* [28] reported that in PGGN, the maximum diameter of 10mm is differentiated as non-invasive, A specific critical point between venereal and invasive diseases [29]. Goo *et al.* [30] studied 94 cases of pure ground-glass nodules. It was suggested that the critical value of infiltration lesions before and after was 10.5mm, and the sensitivity and specificity of diagnosis were 86.30%, 61.90%, respectively; Liu *et al.* [31] conducted a THREE-DIMENSIONAL quantitative analysis of 105 cases of pure ground-glass nodules, showing infiltration lesions before and after. The critical value of the maximum cross-section length diameter was 11.5mm, the diagnostic sensitivity and specificity were 63.3% and 76.0%, respectively. When the critical value was reduced to 10.5mm, the sensitivity and specificity were 76.6% and 62.0%, respectively.

3.5. Real Proportion

The higher the proportion of solid components in the ground glass nodules, the higher the degree of malignancy [32], especially for persistent grinding. Vitreous nodule shadow, when the solid component of > is 50%, often indicates a high possibility of malignancy [33]. AAH is often seen on HRCT images. It usually presents as a very light, pure ground-glass density nodule with a clear boundary, round/quasi-round, and constant diameter of 5 mm or less [34].

AIS and MIA are mostly 5m-30mm in diameter in pure ground-glass nodules [30], but a few are also Partial solid nodules. IA appears mostly as mixed ground-glass nodules and rarely as pure ground-glass knots Section. Lee *et al.* [13] believed that the proportion of solid components in preinvasive lesions (AAH and AIS) was (29.6±18.1) %. The proportion of solid components in MIA and IA was lower (56.7±26.6) %, and 28.6% was differential. Godoy *et al.* [35] divided 241 cases of ground-glass nodules into the infiltrating group and the non-infiltrating or micro-infiltrating group. The difference between solid components was statistically significant. Song [36] believed that when the CT threshold was -250 HU. And -300 HU was used to determine the volume of solid components in the ground glass nodule, corresponding to the solid proportion bounds. The limit value is 1.10% and 6.14%. If the value is lower than or equal to the limit value, it is a pure ground-glass nodule; otherwise, it is part of solid nodules.

3.6. Doubling Time

Subsequently, Time DT is often referred to as the time required to double the volume of tumors, as well as Called Volume Doubling Time VDT, and the units are usually calculated by a few days. Subsequently, the use of mass Time MDT was proposed by scholars. Doubling time to some extent reflects the growth pattern and speed of tumor cells, the degree of activity, the infiltration intensity, and the doubling time of pulmonary nodules. Too fast and too slow are often indicated as benign lesions [37]. According to the Consensus of Chinese experts on the diagnosis and treatment of pulmonary nodules (2018 edition), For pure ground-glass nodule ≤5mm, 6,12...After a month's follow-up, > 5mm was taken, 3,12...Monthly follow-up, For mixed ground-glass nodules ≤8mm, take 3,6,12,24,12...Follow-up, > 8mm followed for 3 months Visit, if the continued increase can be treated with surgery. Hasegawa's [33] performed a 3-year follow-up of 82 patients with malignant disease. Analysis of pulmonary nodules showed that the average doubling time of solid nodules was the shortest, 149 days. The average doubling time of density nodules was 457 days, and the doubling time of density nodules of pure ground glass was 813 days. Oda *et al* [38] studied the average multiplication of pure ground-glass nodules and mixed ground-glass nodules based on the 3D volume measurement method. The time was (628.5±404.2) days and (276.9±155.9) days, respectively.

3.7. Compactness and Sphericity Degree

Sphericity degree (SD) refers to the ratio of the surface area of the sphere with the same volume as the lesion [39], that is, in shape. The closer it is to the shape of the ball, the closer its SD is to 1, which is also called SD and circle in relevant literature reports. Degree, roundness, roundness, *etc*. The larger the SD is, the closer the lesion is to the roundness, which is malignant to a certain extent. The lower the probability, the smaller the SD, indicating the more irregular shape of the lesion and the relative likelihood of malignancy. The compactness mainly reflects the concavity of the edge of the lesion [40], and the calculation formula is as follows:

$$F = 4\ PI\ A/P$$

Where P is the perimeter of the contour of the lesion, A is the area of the lesion, the compactness of the circle F=1, and the more complex the edge of the lesion.

Roughly, the flatter the shape, the less compact it is. Usually, the radiologist looks directly at the shape and edge of the lesion by the naked eye. It is benign and malignant, and the naked eye can only determine the general shape of the lesion, such as round or quasi-round, whether the edge of the lesion spans. Ground glass nodules are mostly early. Stage I lung cancer is often round, and its edge features are not obvious, it is difficult to directly judge by the naked eye. AI-based on deep learning has two advantages in feature extraction of lesions. With a holistic view, it is more accurate to measure the circumference, volume, surface area, and diameter of lesions in a three-dimensional space on the one hand. On the other hand, it displays the detailed features of the lesion, such as some subtle contour inflection points. In these aspects, AI has obvious advantages and is benign and malignant to ground-glass nodules. This judgment has important reference value.

4. OUTLOOK AND PROGRESS

Lung cancer is the leading cause of cancer morbidity and mortality in the world, and the early manifestation of lung adenocarcinoma is often ground glass. As the application of AI and algorithms are becoming more popular and accurate, AI will soon become the routine screening method of radiologists and important assistance in the detection of early lung cancer. With the rapid development of deep learning technology, AI is used to find the lung ground-glass nodules, CT value, maximum surface area, volume, 3D length and diameter, the proportion of compactness, doubling time, compactness, and the proportion of the tumor. In the future, the use of AI in healthcare will be more extensive and in-depth, resulting in the early pathological diagnosis of pulmonary grinding glass nodules in predicting the suitable time for surgery. It can also help the clinicians to assess the prognosis and survival time for the patients. In recent years, with big data and Artificial Intelligence (AI) based on deep learning and the rapid rise of advanced technologies, AI has been developing rapidly in all fields [41 - 45], especially in the diagnosis of pulmonary nodules. The application of section detection can help physicians quickly detect pulmonary nodules and predict their benign and malignant risk at an early stage.

CONSENT FOR PUBLICATION

Not Applicable.

CONFLICT OF INTEREST

The author confirms that this chapter contents have no conflict of interest.

ACKNOWLEDGEMENT

Declared none.

ABBREVIATION

AI   artificial intelligence

GGN   ground-glass nodule

PGGN   pure ground-glass nodules

mGGN   mixed ground-glass nodules

mGGN   part-solid nodules

PACS   Picture Archiving and Communication Systems

IASLC the International Association for the Study of Lung Cancer

ERS   European Respiratory Society

ATS   American Thoracic Society

AAH   atypical adenomatous hyperplasia

AIS   adenocarcinoma *in situ*

MIA   minimally invasive adenocarcinoma

IAC   invasive adenocarcinoma

HRCT High-Resolution CT

LDCT Low-dose computed tomography

SN   solid nodules

SD   Sphericity degree

NCCN National Comprehensive Cancer Network

CNN   Convolutional Neural Network

DT   Doubling time

VDT   volume doubling time

MDT   mass doubling time

REFERENCES

[1]   Alom MZ, *et al.* The history began from alexnet: A comprehensive survey on deep learning approaches 2018.

[2]   Grigorescu S, Trasnea B, Cocias T, Macesanu G. A survey of deep learning techniques for autonomous driving. J Field Robot 2020; 37(3): 362-86.
[http://dx.doi.org/10.1002/rob.21918]

[3]   Nguyen G, Dlugolinsky S, Bobák M, Tran V, García ÁL, Heredia I, *et al.* Machine Learning and Deep Learning frameworks and libraries for large-scale data mining: a survey. Artif Intell Rev 2019; 52(1): 77-124.
[http://dx.doi.org/10.1007/s10462-018-09679-z]

[4]   Hinton GE, Salakhutdinov RR. Reducing the dimensionality of data with neural networks. Science 2006; 313(5786): 504-7.
[http://dx.doi.org/10.1126/science.1127647] [PMID: 16873662]

[5]   Benedetti M, Lloyd E, Sack S, Fiorentini M. Parameterized quantum circuits as machine learning models. Quantum Science and Technology 2019; 4(4): 043001.
[http://dx.doi.org/10.1088/2058-9565/ab4eb5]

[6]   Behzadi-Khormouji H, Rostami H, Salehi S, *et al.* Deep learning, reusable and problem-based architectures for detection of consolidation on chest X-ray images. Comput Methods Programs Biomed 2020; 185(3): 105162.
[http://dx.doi.org/10.1016/j.cmpb.2019.105162] [PMID: 31715332]

[7]   Dunjko V, Briegel HJ. Machine learning & artificial intelligence in the quantum domain: a review of recent progress. Rep Prog Phys 2018; 81(7): 074001.
[http://dx.doi.org/10.1088/1361-6633/aab406] [PMID: 29504942]

[8] Gavrishchaka V, Senyukova O, Koepke M. Synergy of physics-based reasoning and machine learning in biomedical applications: towards unlimited deep learning with limited data. Advances in Physics 2019; 4(1): 1582361.
[http://dx.doi.org/10.1080/23746149.2019.1582361]

[9] Xu XY, Lin N, Li YM, Zhi C, Shen H. Expression of HAb18G/CD147 and its localization correlate with the progression and poor prognosis of non-small cell lung cancer. Pathol Res Pract 2013; 209(6): 345-52.
[http://dx.doi.org/10.1016/j.prp.2013.02.015] [PMID: 23602236]

[10] Leithner D, Wichmann JL, Mahmoudi S, *et al.* Diagnostic yield of 90-kVp low-tube-voltage carotid and intracerebral CT-angiography: effects on radiation dose, image quality and diagnostic performance for the detection of carotid stenosis. Br J Radiol 2018; 91(1086): 20170927-.
[http://dx.doi.org/10.1259/bjr.20170927] [PMID: 29493282]

[11] Chang B, Hwang JH, Choi YH, *et al.* Natural history of pure ground-glass opacity lung nodules detected by low-dose CT scan. Chest 2013; 143(1): 172-8.
[http://dx.doi.org/10.1378/chest.11-2501] [PMID: 22797081]

[12] Xu DM, van Klaveren RJ, de Bock GH, *et al.* Role of baseline nodule density and changes in density and nodule features in the discrimination between benign and malignant solid indeterminate pulmonary nodules. Eur J Radiol 2009; 70(3): 492-8.
[http://dx.doi.org/10.1016/j.ejrad.2008.02.022] [PMID: 18417311]

[13] Lee HY. Pure ground-glass opacity neoplastic lung nodules: histopathology imaging and management. Am J Roenlgen 2014; 202(3): w224-33.

[14] Lee HY, Choi YL, Lee Ks, *et al.* Pure ground-glass opacity neoplastic lung nodules histopathology imaging and management. Am J Roenlgen01 2014; 202(3): w224-33.

[15] Peng M, Li Z, Hu H, *et al.* Pulmonary ground-glass nodules diagnose: mean change rate of peak CT number as a discriminative factor of pathology during a follow-up/ Br J Radiol 2016; 89(1058): 120150556.

[16] Horton EB, Folland CK, Parker DE. The changing incidence of extremes in worldwide and central England temperatures to the end of the twentieth century. Clim Change 2001; 50(3): 267-95.
[http://dx.doi.org/10.1023/A:1010603629772]

[17] Ohtsuka T, Watanabe K, Kaji M, Naruke T, Suemasu K. A clinicopathological study of resected pulmonary nodules with focal pure ground-glass opacity. Eur J Cardiothorac Surg 2006; 30(1): 160-3.
[http://dx.doi.org/10.1016/j.ejcts.2006.03.058] [PMID: 16723239]

[18] Travis WD, Asamura H, Bankier AA, Beasley MB, Detterbeck F, Flieder DB, *et al.* The IASLC lung cancer staging project: proposals for coding T categories for subsolid nodules and assessment of tumor size in part-solid tumors in the forthcoming eighth edition of the TNM classification of lung cancer. J Thoracic Oncology 2016; 11(8): 1204-23.

[19] Han L, Zhang P, Wang Y, *et al.* CT quantitative parameters to predict the invasiveness of lung pure ground-glass nodules(pGGNs). Clinical Radiology 2018; 73(5): 504.el-7.

[20] Ma SH, Le HB, Jia BH, *et al.* Peripheral pulmonary nodules: relationship between multi-slice spiral CT perfusion imaging and tumor angiogenesis and VEGF expression. BMC Cancer 2008; 8(1): 186.
[http://dx.doi.org/10.1186/1471-2407-8-186] [PMID: 18590539]

[21] Schaefer JF, Vollmar J, Schick F, *et al.* Solitary pulmonary nodules: dynamic contrast-enhanced MR imaging--perfusion differences in malignant and benign lesions. Radiology 2004; 232(2): 544-53.
[http://dx.doi.org/10.1148/radiol.2322030515] [PMID: 15215548]

[22] McNitt-Gray MF, Wyckoff N, Sayre JW, Goldin JG, Aberle DR. The effects of co-occurrence matrix based texture parameters on the classification of solitary pulmonary nodules imaged on computed tomography. Comput Med Imaging Graph 1999; 23(6): 339-48.
[http://dx.doi.org/10.1016/S0895-6111(99)00033-6] [PMID: 10634146]

[23]   Gupta NC, Frank AR, Dewan NA, *et al.* Solitary pulmonary nodules: detection of malignancy with PET with 2-[F-18]-fluoro-2-deoxy-D-glucose. Radiology 1992; 184(2): 441-4.
[http://dx.doi.org/10.1148/radiology.184.2.1620844] [PMID: 1620844]

[24]   Chae HD, Park CM, Park SJ, Lee SM, Kim KG, Goo JM. Computerized texture analysis of persistent part-solid ground-glass nodules: differentiation of preinvasive lesions from invasive pulmonary adenocarcinomas. Radiology 2014; 273(1): 285-93.
[http://dx.doi.org/10.1148/radiol.14132187] [PMID: 25102296]

[25]   Yankelevitz DF, Reeves AP, Kostis WJ, Zhao B, Henschke CI. Small pulmonary nodules: volumetrically determined growth rates based on CT evaluation. Radiology 2000; 217(1): 251-6.
[http://dx.doi.org/10.1148/radiology.217.1.r00oc33251] [PMID: 11012453]

[26]   Petrick N, Kim HJG, Clunie D, *et al.* Comparison of 1D, 2D, and 3D nodule sizing methods by radiologists for spherical and complex nodules on thoracic CT phantom images. Acad Radiol 2014; 21(1): 30-40.
[http://dx.doi.org/10.1016/j.acra.2013.09.020] [PMID: 24331262]

[27]   Naidich DP, Bankier AA, MacMahon H, *et al.* Recommendations for the management of subsolid pulmonary nodules detected at CT: a statement from the Fleischner Society. Radiology 2013; 266(1): 304-17.
[http://dx.doi.org/10.1148/radiol.12120628] [PMID: 23070270]

[28]   Lee HY. Pure ground-glass opacity neoplastic lung nodules: histopathology imaging and management. Am Roenlgen 01 2014; 202(3): w224-33.2014;

[29]   Lee SM, Park CM, Goo JM, Lee HJ, Wi JY, Kang CH. Invasive pulmonary adenocarcinomas *versus* preinvasive lesions appearing as ground-glass nodules: differentiation by using CT features. Radiology 2013; 268(1): 265-73.
[http://dx.doi.org/10.1148/radiol.13120949] [PMID: 23468575]

[30]   Goo JM, Park CM, Lee HJ. Ground-glass nodules on chest CT as imaging biomarkers in the management of lung adenocarcinoma. AJR Am J Roentgenol 2011; 196(3): 533-43.
[http://dx.doi.org/10.2214/AJR.10.5813] [PMID: 21343494]

[31]   Liu L, Wu N, Tang W, *et al.* The morphological changes of bronchovascular bundles within subsolid nodules on HRCT correlate with the new IASLC classification of adenocarcinoma. Clin Radiol 2018; 73(6): 542-8.
[http://dx.doi.org/10.1016/j.crad.2017.12.009] [PMID: 29329734]

[32]   Yaguchi A, Okazakt T, Takeguchi T. Semi-automated segmentation of solid and GGO nudules in lung CT images using vessel-likelihood derived from local foreground structure. Medical Imaging 2015: Computer-Aided Diagnosis 2015.

[33]   Ohde Y, Nagai K, Yoshida J, *et al.* The pmponion of consolidation to ground-glass opacity on high resolution CT is a good predictor fbr distinguishing the population of non-invasive peripheral adenocarcinoma. Imng Cancer 2003; 42(3): 303-10.

[34]   Chang B, Hwang JH, Choi YH, *et al.* Natural history of pure ground-glass opacity lung nodules detected by low-dose CT scan. Chest 2013; 143(1): 172-8.
[http://dx.doi.org/10.1378/chest.11-2501] [PMID: 22797081]

[35]   Godoy MC, Naidich DP. Overview and strategic management of subsolid pulmonary nodules. J Thorac Imaging 2012; 27(4): 240-8.
[http://dx.doi.org/10.1097/RTI.0b013e31825d515b] [PMID: 22847591]

[36]   Song YS, Park CM, Park SJ, Lee SM, Jeon YK, Goo JM. Volume and mass doubling times of persistent pulmonary subsolid nodules detected in patients without known malignancy. Radiology 2014; 273(1): 276-84.
[http://dx.doi.org/10.1148/radiol.14132324] [PMID: 24927472]

[37]   Song YS, Park CM, Park SJ, Lee SM, Jeon YK, Goo JM. Volume and mass doubling times of

persistent pulmonary subsolid nodules detected in patients without known malignancy. Radiology 2014; 273(1): 276-84.
[http://dx.doi.org/10.1148/radiol.14132324] [PMID: 24927472]

[38]   Oda S, Awai K, Murao K, *et al.* Volume-doubling time of pulmonary nodules with ground glass opacity at multidetector CT: Assessment with computer-aided three-dimensional volumetry. Acad Radiol 2011; 18(1): 63-9.
[http://dx.doi.org/10.1016/j.acra.2010.08.022] [PMID: 21145028]

[39]   Kar S, Das Sharma K, Maitra M. Adaptive weighted aggregation in Group Improvised Harmony Search for lung nodule classification. J Exp Theor Artif Intell 2020; 32(2): 219-42.
[http://dx.doi.org/10.1080/0952813X.2019.1647561]

[40]   Chien KCC. Automated lung screening system of multiple pathological targets in multislice CT. 2011.

[41]   Hu Q, Yang J, Qin P, Fong S. Towards a context-free machine universal grammar (CF-MUG) in natural language processing. IEEE Access 2020; 8: 165111-29.
[http://dx.doi.org/10.1109/ACCESS.2020.3022674]

[42]   Yang J, Huang SG, Tang R. Broad learning with attribute selection for rheumatoid arthritis. IEEE International Conference on Systems, Man and Cybernetics (SMC). Toronto: IEEE 2020.

[43]   Hu Q, Yang J, Qin P, Fong S, Guo J. Could or could not of Grid-Loc: grid BLE structure for indoor localisation system using machine learning. Serv Oriented Comput Appl 2020.
[http://dx.doi.org/10.1007/s11761-020-00292-z]

[44]   Yang J, Fong S, Li T. Attribute reduction based on multi-objective decomposition-ensemble optimizer with rough set and entropy. International Conference on Data Mining Workshops (ICDMW). IEEE 2019; pp. 673-80.

[45]   Huang S, Yang J, Fong S, Zhao Q. Artificial intelligence in cancer diagnosis and prognosis: Opportunities and challenges. Cancer Lett 2020; 471: 61-71.
[http://dx.doi.org/10.1016/j.canlet.2019.12.007] [PMID: 31830558]

Current and Future Application of Artificial Intelligence, 2021, 109-131   **109**

CHAPTER 9

Development of Artificial Intelligence in Imaging and Pathology

Gang Liu[1] and Tao Qi[2,*]

[1] *Tourism College, Hainan University, 58 Renmin Road, Haikou, Hainan Province, 570228, P. R. China*

[2] *Department of Radiation Oncology, 986 Hospital of People's Liberation Army Air Force, Xi'an, Shaan Xi, P. R. China*

Abstract: Abstract: Artificial intelligence technology is frontier technology as the interaction and cooperation between AI, and different disciplines can bring great opportunities and impetus to the development in social, scientific, and technological progress. This chapter included AI in imaging, pathology, and development in pathological diagnosis. With the continuous progress of society and science, AI technology has penetrated all aspects of human production and life, greatly promoting the liberation of productivity and the change in human lifestyle. Among them, the medical field is the one that has been significantly changed. The development and integration of the two disciplines have brought great changes to the development of healthcare systems across the globe. AI technology has been widely used in the field of medical treatment, including medical education, medical imaging, pathology, diagnostics, medical robotics, medical data management, molecular tumor research, *etc.* However, with time, the disadvantages of AI have been gradually exposed, and this historic cross-border cooperation also faces many challenges.

Keywords: Artificial intelligence, Digital diagnosis, Digital pathology, Imaging, Pathology.

1. INTRODUCTION

The analysis of medical images and pathology is an important area of application for deep learning. It is possible to extract and learn image and pathology features from large-scale data [1]. When the computational efficiency has increased dramatically, it can extract useful information from massive amounts of data. One basic model of deep learning is Convolutional Neural Networks (CNN), an algori-

---
* **Corresponding author Tao Qi:** Department of Radiation Oncology, 986 Hospital of People's Liberation Army Air Force, Xi'an, Shaan Xi, P. R. China; E-mail: 309384509@qq.com.

Shigao Huang and Jie Yang (Eds.)

thm that has been applied in many medical imaging and pathology analyses. We are seeing a proliferation of task-specific AI applications around us that can rival and occasionally surpass human intelligence [2]. AI imaging plays an important role in AI medicine, and a large number of relevant technical research literature have been published.

The concept similar to the combination of AI and medical imaging was first proposed by Lusted LB in 1960, who believed that symbolic logic and probabilistic reasoning had significant value in the transmission of medical diagnosis [3], which could be regarded as the early model of medical AI. 90% of the medical data are from medical imaging, and the current medical imaging data in China is increasing at an annual rate of 30% [4]. Some scholars believe that the combination of medical imaging and AI technology is the most promising field [5].

2. AI IMAGING

2.1. Overview of AI Imaging

Historically, in radiology practice, experienced physicians have used medical images for visual assessment to detect, describe, and monitor the disease. AI is good at automatically identifying complex patterns in imaging data and providing quantitative rather than qualitative assessment of radiographic features [6]. "Artificial intelligence + medical images" refers to the classification, segmentation, registration, fusion, and retrieval of medical images using deep learning methods, to assist doctors in completing diagnosis and treatment [4, 7].

With the continuous development in imaging and AI, the image omics concept proposed by scholars took the lead in 2012 by Lambin [8] to extract large data samples and the in-depth mining, or data analysis, and interpretation, to find out additional implicit information in the image, through the analysis of original data to assist practitioner and guide the clinician's decision.

The analysis process includes:

Image acquisition: Image acquisition through CT, MRI, PET, and other image scanning methods.

Image segmentation: The abnormal tissues or specific anatomical tissues in the image are divided into one or more regions of interest.

Feature extraction: Image features, mainly including strength, shape, texture, location, and other features.

Quantitative analysis: The statistical analysis of the above characteristics, the commonly used analysis methods include repeated measurement reliability analysis, principal component analysis, correlation analysis, and random forest.

Model construction: A prediction and classification model based on image omics features is established through machine learning (deep learning) [4, 9].

2.2. Research Progress of AI Imaging

In the fields of pulmonary nodules, renal tumors, radiotherapy, breast cancer, diabetic retinopathy screening, AI has made many achievements [10]. Some scholars detected molybdenum target X-ray lesions (mass, breast and axillary lymph nodes, calcification) through AI and found that the sensitivity was 95.6%, 74.1%, and 72.5%, and the false-positive rates were 4.6%, 34.8%, and 37.7%, respectively. Also, for bi-RADS 2 and 3, the sensitivity was 85.6% and 68.2%, respectively, and the false-positive rate was 14.3% and 31.7%, respectively. Calcification is less effective than lumps and lymph nodes in the breast, and it may be related to factors such as the density of the breast gland, fat accumulation, and the pixel size of the camera. The above-mentioned studies have shown that AI diagnostic technology is competitive with human doctors in indicating sensitivity and false positives. It will make AI a hope and an auxiliary reference tool for clinicians. AI combined with the clinical environment can reduce the misdiagnosis rate and improve the diagnosis effect [11].

AI plays an important auxiliary role in CT scanning for radiologists. The conventional chest CT model has about 300 images, and manual reading is adopted. A trained doctor needs 3-5 minutes on average and is prone to omission. The low-dose CT+AI method can comprehensively screen the pulmonary nodules in the chest of patients and intuitively display the location, size, composition, and other basic information of each node within 3-5 seconds. In the field of optometry, based on the deep study of diabetic retinopathy, an artificially intelligent diagnosis system can display the severity of the fundus lesions [12].

Some scholars retrospectively collected 39 patients with hyperfast angiomyolipoma and 41 patients with renal clear cell carcinoma. Tumor-related features were extracted from the enhanced ABDOMINAL CT image and combined with these features to distinguish renal clear cell carcinoma from hyperfast angiomyolipoma, with an accuracy rate of 76.6% [13]. SkinVision, developed by Dutch researchers, can diagnose skin melanomas with picture recognition with an accuracy rate of 73 percent and is expected to alert users to suspicious moles or consult a doctor as soon as possible. In the skin cancer diagnosis project studied by the Research team of Stanford University, the accuracy of AI diagnosis has reached 91%, which is equal to that of artificial diagnosis [14].

Dermatology researchers in China are also collecting and collating basic data and formulating industry-related technical standards to make unremitting efforts for the development of AI skin imaging diagnosis technology. Tim Lustberg and others, based on the outline of the atlas (AC) and deep learning outline (DLC), automatically used time frame and manual frame method and found that lung cancer OAR frame automatic method compared with an artificial method can save time 7.8-10 minutes [15].

For OAR framing, some scholars also retrospectively analyzed 10 experimental reports on OAR framing of head and neck tumors and found that the results were contradictory [16]. The automatic framing method saved 59% of the reports, while some cases took 15.7% more time. Daniel A. Orringer *et al.* [17] created virtual hemagglutinin - eosin staining slides to diagnose surgical specimens by simulating the Raman histology (SRH) image processing method and found that pathological diagnosis was the gold standard, and the consistency of the two was detected by $0.89(p = 0.031)$, the accuracy of this method is more than 92%. Compared with the time-consuming and laborious method of traditional intraoperative histopathological section diagnosis, the new AI method is more simple and effective and also avoids delaying the decision-making time of tumor resection.

Zhang *et al.* [18] showed that lymph node B ultrasonic examination under the computer-aided technology declared that the physician performance was improved obviously from 0.843 to 0.896 $(p = 0.031)$.

These results showed that computer-assisted diagnosis could improve the performance of radiologists (especially inexperienced radiologists) in the ultrasound evaluation of cervical lymph nodes and reduce the differences among radiologists.

3. PATHOLOGY

Disadvantages of traditional pathological tissue sections, such as difficulty in the preservation and poor information sharing, have increasingly promoted the development of digital electronic slice technology. Digital pathology is character-ized by ease in preservation and management, convenient transmission and sharing, high definition, *etc.*, and has irreplaceable advantages in pathology teaching, remote consultation, scientific research, and development, *etc.*

On this basis, modern pathological diagnostics is moving towards the direction of large-scale digitization of microscope. Khomfoi *et al.* [19] concluded that artificial intelligence (AI) technology brings great potential to the evaluation of immune-histo-chemical slices through the data analysis of the Her2 simulation competition. The medical mammary matrix microenvironment is a key factor in the occurrence, development, and metastasis of breast cancer. Ehteshami Bejnordi B *et al.* found that the detection of morphological changes of the substrate by light microscope was subjective and non-quantitative, and the algorithm based on a deep convolutional neural network is to only evaluate the substrate and might be helpful for classification of breast biopsy and understanding and evaluating the biological characteristics of breast lesions [20]. Numerous studies have shown that ai pathology techniques can sometimes save doctors' time and free them from tedious, unskilled work. Dordea *et al.* [21] used free, open-source software CP and CPA to automatically quantify retinal ganglion cells in rats [22]. The authors found that automated methods made their analysis about 10 times faster. Diem *et al.* [20] used automatic image analysis to count CD4+ and CD8+T cells and showed that even in images with high cell density, automatic counting was about 10 minutes faster than manual counting. It is worth noting that automatic counting allows for faster processing and analysis of samples, and the saved image can be reanalyzed multiple times and this is a very important advantage in some areas. Macedo N.D *et al.* [23] found in their study that automatic image analysis has great clinical, diagnostic, and research potential, and provides a new quantitative ability, thus adding quantitative numerical information to most qualitative diagnostic methods.

3.1. Exploration of AI in Pathological Diagnosis

In March 2017, scientists from Google Brain, Google, and Verily Life Science tested 130 pathological sections of breast cancer lymph node metastasis lesions by using AI technology constructed by a recurrent neural network.

Meanwhile, a pathologist took 30 hours to run the same test, and the AI achieved an accuracy rate of 88.5 percent, while the pathologist's accuracy rate was only 73.3 percent. In June 2016, at the international symposium on biomedical imaging, from Beth Israel Deaconess Medical Center (Beth Israel Deaconess Medical Center, BIDMC) developed a team of researchers at Harvard Medical school based on the deep study of the AI technology, the pathologist analysis, and AI, automatic calculation of diagnostic methods, the combination of sentinel lymph node metastasis of breast cancer diagnosis accuracy increased to 99. 5%.

Dr. Beck then founded a diagnostic technology company called Path AI to develop and apply AI technology to help pathologists make diagnoses faster and more accurately. In March 2017, Philips, a Dutch multinational electronics company, announced a partnership with the company. Deep Care is a Chinese technology company that uses AI and deep learning technologies for medical image recognition and screening.

3.2. Grading of Renal Clear Cell Carcinoma

Yeh *et al.* [24] used WSI to locate the characteristic areas in sections of 39 patients with different grades of renal clear cell carcinoma and then performed Fuhrman grading based on features such as the size of the tumor nucleus. Analysis shows that by the size, he tried to distinguish high-level (III and IV level), and low level (I and II) tumor of the false positive rate of 0. 2, the true positive rate of 1. 0 (area under the curve is AUC = 0. 97).

3. 3. Segmentation of Neoplastic Glandular Structure in Colorectal Cancer

About 80% of colorectal cancer develops from colorectal adenomas. The structural and morphological changes of neoplastic glands may predict the prognosis of patients. Therefore, an automated method to quantify the morphology of the glands is the key to solving this problem. Glands are irregular clumps of body shape structure, and characterized by pathological slice thickness and evenness, the existence of impurities and dyeing depth and digital image noise image heterogeneity, the influence of factors such as deep learning to use the convolution neural network for the classification of the presence of glands, and then use segmentation algorithm segmentation of a single gland, unstable factors to the outside to minimize the impact of the late diagnosis [25].

3.4. Detection of MYCO Bacterium Tuberculosis in Special Staining

Xiong *et al.* [26] established a convolutional neural network model of Mycobacterium tuberculosis AI(TB-AI). Forty-five samples (30 positive cases and 15 negative cases) were used to train the model. After training the neural network model, 201 samples (108 positive cases and 93 negative cases) were collected as test sets and used to examine TB-AI. Through the pathologist, by dual diagnosis with digital slides, TB-AI achieved a sensitivity of 97.94% and specificity of 83.65% for the detection of mycobacterium tuberculosis in special staining.

3.5. Determination of Proliferating Cells in Cervical Epithelial Lesions

The proliferation of tumor cells in intraepithelial neoplasia, and high-grade intraepithelial neoplasia reflects normal cervical tissue and low-level cervix by expression of P16 and KI-67.The. Training an end-to-end network (N) -net or Whole Image (WI) -net) enabled them to predict the pixel value of molecular markers in the Whole glass slide Image of immunostaining. The results showed that the coincidence rate between the automatic determination results and the manual determination results obtained by the pathologist (positive p16, positive KI-67, positive P16 and KI-67, and negative P16 and KI-67) reached 96% [27]. The expression of Her2 is a key part of the diagnostic evaluation in invasive breast cancer and is recognized as an important clinical issue Predictors. Automated Her2 scoring based on AI can reduce the differences caused by the subjectivity of visual scoring. In a comparison of the results of Her2 in 86 cases of invasive breast cancer, the competition algorithm showed a greater advantage by analyzing the HE and IHC full-slide images to predict the expression results, demonstrating the great potential of the automatic algorithm in assisting pathologists to perform IHC objective scores.

4. THE EXPLORATION OF AI IN TUMOR PROGNOSTIC JUDGMENT

4.1. Prediction of Survival in Patients with Non-small Cell Lung Cancer and Breast Cancer

Kun-Hsing Yu and colleagues [28] (Stanford University, USA) used the genome of 2186 patients with lung adenocarcinoma and squamous cell carcinoma tissue pathology slice and a database of 294 images from Stanford tissue microarray. They used image analysis software and 9879 figure-like quantitative features for extracting machine learning software for these images then they developed to identify the classifier of tumor cells, used to distinguish lung adenocarcinoma and squamous cell carcinoma, and predict survival. The data showed that the classifier was effective in distinguishing malignant tumors from adjacent normal tissues (mean area under the subject operating characteristic curve, AUC = 0.81) and was able to distinguish between two different types of NSCLC(AUC > 0.75) [29 - 38].

Furthermore, it is also effective in predicting long-term survival for stage I adenocarcinoma (log-rank P = 0.0023) and squamous cell carcinoma (log-rank P = 0.023) [39]. Beck *et al* [40]. from Harvard Medical School used 248 breast cancer patients from the Netherlands Cancer Institute (NKI) and 328 breast cancer patients from Vancouver General Hospital (VGH) as pathological images and selected a total of 671 (NKI) and 615 (VGH) breast cancer WSI for analysis. In my previous study [41], we used AI for the prognosis regarding brain metastasis from NSCLC. Fig. (**1**) described the importance of ranking comparison of cancer features in patients for different weights in the MIRSPSO algorithm. Besides, Fig. (**1**) showed that primary tumor control was the most important in patients. The levels of significance for each feature are visualized in the form of the heat map.

Using an integrated pathway system they independently developed to measure a large number of image features (6,642) from the breast cancer epithelium and stroma, they constructed a prognostic model based on image features to predict 5-year survival in patients [42]. In the end, 11 features were found to be most closely related to prognosis, among which 8 were from epithelial cells and 3 were from stroma, and the correlation between the features of these 3 stroma and 5-year survival rate was stronger than that of epithelial features in the model. These results suggest that matrix morphology may be an important prognostic determinant of breast cancer that has not been previously concerned [34].

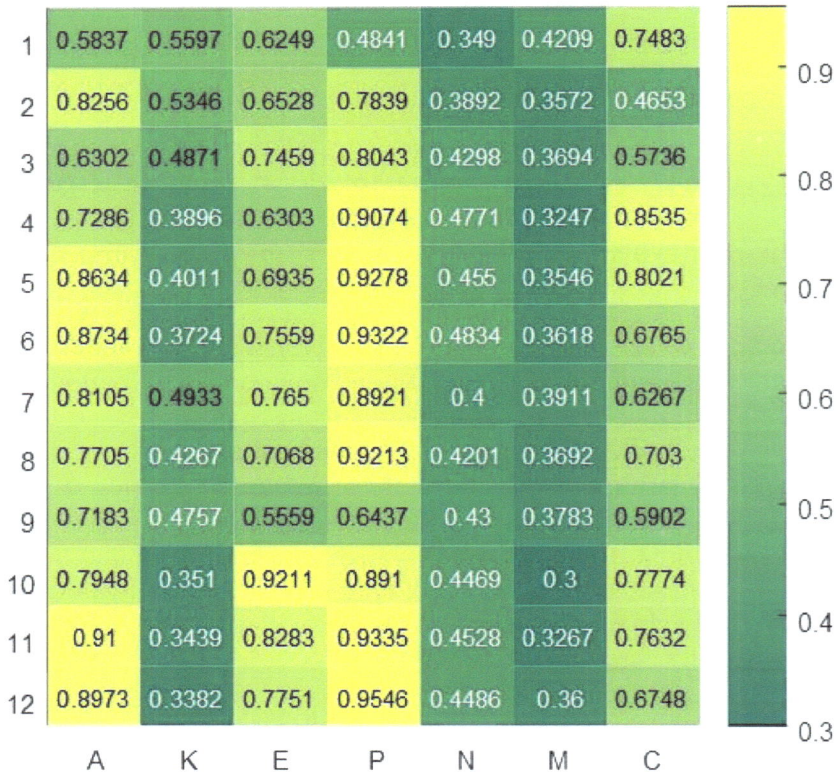

	A	K	E	P	N	M	C
1	0.5837	0.5597	0.6249	0.4841	0.349	0.4209	0.7483
2	0.8256	0.5346	0.6528	0.7839	0.3892	0.3572	0.4653
3	0.6302	0.4871	0.7459	0.8043	0.4298	0.3694	0.5736
4	0.7286	0.3896	0.6303	0.9074	0.4771	0.3247	0.8535
5	0.8634	0.4011	0.6935	0.9278	0.455	0.3546	0.8021
6	0.8734	0.3724	0.7559	0.9322	0.4834	0.3618	0.6765
7	0.8105	0.4933	0.765	0.8921	0.4	0.3911	0.6267
8	0.7705	0.4267	0.7068	0.9213	0.4201	0.3692	0.703
9	0.7183	0.4757	0.5559	0.6437	0.43	0.3783	0.5902
10	0.7948	0.351	0.9211	0.891	0.4469	0.3	0.7774
11	0.91	0.3439	0.8283	0.9335	0.4528	0.3267	0.7632
12	0.8973	0.3382	0.7751	0.9546	0.4486	0.36	0.6748

Fig. (1). Heat map declared that the predictive performance (AUC) of the relationship between cancer features and importance degree in patients. P: Primary tumor control was the most important degree in patients. This fig was from Huang *et al.*, Cancers, 2019 [43].

4.2. Predicting whether Patients with Stage T1 Colon Cancer need Additional Radical Surgery

AI can help predict whether patients with stage T1 colon cancer (CRC) need additional radical surgery after endoscopic resection. Through the SVM algorithm of 590 patients with stage T1 CRC 45 clinical features in-depth study, finally, through the results of 100 patients with stage T1 CRC test, the results compared with the predicted NCCN, ESMO, and JSCCR guidelines, the prediction model of AI can reduce the rate of 8%, 14% and 14% of surgery, and total bilirubin levels, weight, and age [35].

4.3. To Evaluate Postoperative Distant Metastasis in Patients with Esophageal Squamous Cell Carcinoma

The outcomes in the patients with Oesophageal squamous cell carcinoma (OSCC) were evaluated on the following four predictive models of SVM, established to evaluate whether the patients had distant metastasis or not. In addition to T and N stages, 4 other clinic-pathological features and 12 molecular markers were included. Based on 319 cases of postoperative metastasis in patients with OSCC in-depth study, and the testing analysis of 164 patients, finally it is concluded that the optimal combination forecasting is helpful (including four clinical-pathological features: tumor grade, stage and tumor size, tumor differentiation degree, 9: molecular markers cyclin D1, EGFR, HER2 / neu, NF - kB, Integrinb1, Ki - 67, p21Waf1 / Cip1 and uPAR and VEGF).

The data results showed that the SVM-based prediction model had higher sensitivity and accuracy than the TNM staging method proposed by AJCC guidelines to predict postoperative metastasis of OSCC patients [14]. With the integration of WSI and SECOND generation sequencing, the scale and complexity of data will increase. More and more pathologists need to integrate data from multiple sources to produce a more accurate diagnosis and prognostic analysis. Therefore, the multi-mode research and diagnosis prospect of digital pathology combined with the new database is expected by medical workers, especially pathologists. AI relies on its powerful real-time computing ability to make medical research developments in a more in-depth and specific direction, and the leap from qualitative to quantitative opens up infinite possibilities for the development of various disciplines. Kwak *et al.* [36] further extended the prostate histopathological parameters expressed by multi-parameter MRI by associating tissue specimens with multi-parameter MRI, which is likely to improve MRI decision-making and improve the understanding of the source of MRI signal characteristics.

This method can be used for cell selection in tumor genome analysis to further study the correlation between MRI and tumor genomics. Yu K.H *et al.* [37] found that histopathological image classifiers based on quantitative characteristics could successfully predict survival outcomes in patients with lung adenocarcinoma and lung squamous cell carcinoma. This ability is superior to the practice currently being used by pathologists to assess images of tumor grading and staging. The objective characteristics associated with survival also provide insights for histopathological studies. Sickle cell disease (SCD) is a disease of the blood system. The morphology of red blood cells in patients is diverse and has important biomechanical and biological rheological properties. Objective and effective quantification and classification of red blood cell morphology will help to better understand and judge the prognosis of the disease. Some scientists [38] conducted several experiments on the original microscopic image data set (over 7,000 images of single red blood cells) of 8 patients with sickle cell disease and cross-validated oxygenation and deoxygenated red blood cells using a five-fold cross-validation method. The results show that the framework can classify sickle-shaped RBCs in a highly automated manner and provide corresponding shape factor analysis, which can be used in conjunction with deep convolutional neural network (CNN) analysis to improve the persuasive power of prediction. Classification of gastric cancer is an important way to guide the treatment of gastric cancer and predict the survival rate of gastric cancer patients. Sharma *et al.* [38] classified gastric cancer slices through deep learning methods and got a good result. The overall classification accuracy of gastric cancer classification reached 0.6990. Necrotic detection reached 0.8144.

5. DEEP LEARNING IN THE MELANOCYTE TUMOR PATHOLOGICAL DIAGNOSIS

5.1. Deep Learning Development in Pathological Diagnosis

Deep learning is an important breakthrough in the field of AI in the past decade. It has achieved great success in the application of natural language processing, computer vision, speech recognition, and other fields. There are several important reasons for deep learning neural networks to make important breakthroughs: First, the arrival of the era of big data provides a large amount of data for model training, which alleviates the problem of over-fitting in training to a large extent. For example, the ImageNet training set has millions of marked data. Secondly, the rapid development of computer hardware provides it with powerful computing power. A GPU chip can integrate thousands of cores, making it possible to train a large-scale neural network.

The biggest breakthrough in deep learning in computer vision came in 2012, when Hintoth's research team used deep learning networks to win the ImageNet image classification competition, with an accuracy rate of more than 53 percent higher than the second place. This result caused a great surprise in the field of computer vision, which triggered a great upsurge in deep learning. Later, the application of deep learning in the field of medical imaging has become a very hot research direction.

Dermatologist relies on the morphological characteristics of the subject. The skin image is an important means of skin disease diagnosis, so deep learning has broad application prospects in dermatology. In early 2017 at Stanford University, Nature has released the latest breakthrough in the field of skin cancer clinical image diagnosis, which is based on the depth of the InceptioV3 learning network architecture, after 130000 clinical images of skin diseases which can be used to identify cancer diagnosis system [39]. In trials with dermatologists, the system had an accuracy rate of 69.4 percent, compared with about 66 percent for human experts.

In addition to clinical images, deep learning also achieves a very good place in recognition of dermoscopy images. The deep learning model based on ISIC database training is used to identify melanoma and pigmented nevus and is compared with dermatologists. The accuracy of the deep learning algorithm exceeds the average level of doctors [40]. With the popularization of full-fledged digital pathological section images, deep learning has also made a breakthrough in recognition of pathological images. Research shows that the sensitivity and specificity of the deep learning model in the classification of lymph node metastasis of prostate cancer and breast cancer have reached 100% and are between 30-40%. AI and deep learning have achieved very good results in recognition of clinical images, dermoscopy, and pathological images of skin diseases. However, compared with clinical images and dermoscopy images that are also medical images, the application of deep learning in pathological images is much more difficult.

A pathological image is at the magnitude of GB, and its data capacity is more than 10,000 times that of visible light and dermoscopy images, which also brings great challenges to large-scale matrix operations. Therefore, the recognition difficulty of WSI images is much higher than that of visible light images and dermoscopy images. It is for this reason, in the treatment of pathological image when we first put it into image blocks of 256 pixels by, based on the image block to predict [41], and then the predicted results of all the tiles to form the whole pathological image prediction probability heat maps, it reflects the deep learning model to identify the melanoma of the suspected area of the organization.

Based on the predicted probabilistic heat map, the macroscopic features of the suspected area were extracted, and the WSI image was recognized by a random forest classifier to complete the classification of melanoma or pigmented nevus. The pathological diagnosis of melanoma and nevus is a comprehensive judgment combined with low magnification and high magnification, in which the pattern (macroscopic features) is mainly observed under low magnification, and the morphological features of cells (microscopic features) are observed under high magnification [42].

The pathological image input by the DenseNe 169 deep learning model during training is a 256x256 pixel image block [43]. Fig. (2) showed the DenseNe 169 deep learning model to identify the melanoma cells. What the model captures is only the difference between melanoma and pigmented nevus at the image block level, mainly the morphological features of cells. As the above are microscopic characteristics of pathological images, the classification of the deep learning network model at the image block level in the process of prediction is only a process of distinguishing suspected melanoma cells from non-melanoma cells in the microscopic field of view [44].

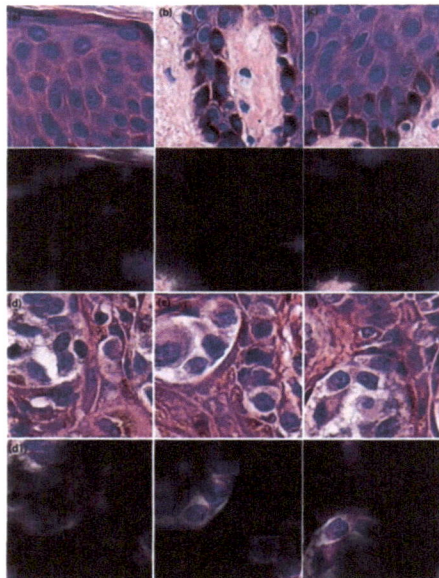

Fig. (2). DenseNet 169 deep learning network model from the sample image block activation regions: al, bl, cl with no highlighted area indicates that deep learning network does not think these areas are focus area, and not in the above extraction melanoma. Characteristic; On the d1, el, f1 melanoma cells in highlighting state region, believed these areas showed that deep learning networks are effective for classification. And then the microscopic image features of melanoma will be extracted from these regions for network learning. The resource was from Ba Wei.,2019 [45].

A final diagnosis based solely on the image block-level (microscopic features) will inevitably lose the important judgment of the distribution pattern of melanoma cells (macroscopic features). So we in the image block-level prediction, prediction probability heat extraction of three different dimensions of eight characteristics (the number of the connected domain, the maximum connected domain area, is the largest circumference of the connected domain, the largest connected domain average probability, the maximum length of the long axis of the connected domain [46], the largest connected domain eccentricity, the maximum connected domain short axis length and maximum rotation Angle of the connected domain), a total of 24 characteristics.

5.2. Diagnostic Melanocyte Benign and Malignant

Based on these features, a random forest classifier is constructed so that the overall recognition process has a comprehensive perception of cell morphology and cell distribution pattern. The classification strategy simulates the process of the comprehensive judgment of the microscopic features combined with the macroscopic features in the pathological diagnosis of melanoma and nevus and achieves a good classification effect in the dichotomous task of melanoma and nevus [46].

Based on our findings, deep learning model of melanocyte source benign and malignant tumors of WSI slice image classification performance is superior to the average of seven doctors, although, under the same sensitivity, specificity, and deep learning model of seven pathology doctors, average specificity was no significant difference, the deep learning model under the same specificity sensitivity is higher than the average sensitivity, seven doctors and AUC of deep learning algorithm should be greater than the average of seven pathology doctor AUC [47].

Pathology is the gold standard for the diagnosis of melanoma, and the early diagnosis of melanoma has an important influence on the treatment of melanoma. However, early accurate diagnosis of melanoma is often difficult to achieve in some underdeveloped medical areas in China. According to the relevant statistics of the National Health and Family Planning Commission, the demand for pathologists in China is 100,000, while the total number of registered pathologists in China is only about 10,000 [48], 9 times as many as the shortage. More serious is the cycle of training of a pathologist who is capable of independently writing a pathology report is generally more than 10 years.

In contrast, training a deep learning model can enable computer algorithms to learn the expertise of industry experts in a short time through a large number of medical cases, so that the computer can achieve similar performance with experts in a certain subdivision field. Therefore, based on the current national conditions in China, the pathological diagnosis system of benign and malignant melanoma based on a deep learning algorithm can be used as a clinical auxiliary diagnostic tool to help pathologists to screen for melanoma. Especially in the underdeveloped areas of medical technology, the significance is even more important. The deep learning neural network can predict pathological images by scanning every region in an all-around way, which is impossible for humans to do [49].

Because over time, the doctor's attention to reducing and fatigue and other objective factors will affect the doctor for pathological observation, and machine learning model will not have this problem, it can perform the tireless work, thus a deep learning model has an effective clinical advantage of a secondary screening tool [50].

Sensitivity, specificity, and AUC cannot reflect the harm caused to patients by missed diagnosis and misdiagnosis. For patients with melanoma cell-derived tumors [51], when misdiagnosis occurs, nevus is misdiagnosed as melanoma, which will cause certain psychological pressure and excessive treatment to the patients but will not cause life threats to the patients. However, when a missed diagnosis occurs, melanoma is treated as pigmented nevus, which may delay the treatment of patients, especially this kind of tumor with a high degree of malignancy, which may pose a threat to patients' lives. The harm caused by missed diagnosis is much higher than that caused by misdiagnosis, so we introduced the evaluation standard of weighted parameters. The experimental results show that the weighted error of the deep learning algorithm is lower than the average level of 7 doctors, indicating that the performance of the deep learning model is better than that of doctors [52].

The mean (± standard deviation) sensitivity and specificity of the 7 pathologists for the classification of benign and malignant melanoma cells were 85.2% (± 3.8%) and 95.6% (± 1.5%), respectively, and the sensitivity fluctuation of the seven pathologists was 86.2%--93.1%. After analysis, among the false-negative results, many doctors classified *in-situ* melanoma and nevus with severe atypical hyperplasia as pigmentation nevus [53].

5.3. Future Progress of AI Diagnosis

In practical clinical work, the diagnosis of typical pigmented nevus and melanoma is relatively clear. But borderline cases can be controversial. This is why we are introducing the mpATH-DX diagnostic criteria [54], which are more consistent with clinical reality. Pathological diagnosis is influenced by subjective factors

[55]. Different doctors have different diagnostic criteria for nevi with moderate atypical hyperplasia and severe atypical hyperplasia/*in-situ* melanoma, which is an important reason for the low sensitivity of some doctors [56].

But deep learning models don't have this problem. A well-trained model that captures the subtle differences between nevi with moderate dysplasia and severe DYSplasia/*in-situ* melanoma will have a more stable and objective output than a doctor [57]. The deep learning model not only gives the classification results but also outputs the basis for the neural network to make the classification, namely probabilistic heat map. The probabilistic heat map showed the severe atypical hyperplasia and melanoma areas judged by the neural network on the WSI image, and most of the predicted areas coexisted with the severe atypical hyperplasia and melanoma areas labeled by the pathologist to be 77.78% [58], indicating that the neural network made classification with accurate identification features. This information can be shared with the pathologist, who can focus on these areas to improve efficiency.

This study also has limitations. The biggest deficiency is that the evaluation of the deep learning model and physician dichotomy level is an approximate simulation process, rather than a real pathological workflow [59]. In practice, pathologists encounter tumors that are mostly melanocyte-derived but are not melanomas, and only a small percentage of these tumors are melanocyte-derived. This is not directly comparable to the complex case mix encountered in clinical practice. In this study, each pathologist provided only 1 H&E staining section to confirm the diagnosis. In the actual clinical environment, pathologists may also do immune poached, combined with the patient's clinical history (age, location, symptoms) to make a comprehensive judgment to improve the accuracy of diagnosis [60]. Besides, because doctors' diagnostic levels are set artificially, they don't have to worry about the serious consequences of missing a diagnosis or misdiagnosing melanoma. These factors may affect the pathologist's diagnostic level. Also, the difference in the inherent difficulty level of the test set will directly affect the deep learning algorithm and the diagnostic efficacy of pathologists. A total of 753 WSI images (639 nevi and 114 melanoma) were used in the training and testing of the deep learning model, but these data are far from sufficient for a mature model with good generalization performance that can be applied to the clinic [61].

Melanoma cells morphological diversity, in addition to the typical epithelioid and spindle, are other rare types including small round and round, polygonal, ballooning, multi-core and dendritic characteristics, such as part of the rare cases does not cover, this means that the deep learning model in training didn't learn these rare morphological features, predicting this part when melanoma may be missing. Future research needs to include more data from multiple centers so that the performance of the system can be further improved. In addition to confirming our results with the help of a larger and more diverse data set, forward-looking studies are needed to address pathologists' acceptance of this new technology.

In summary, our study suggests that a well-trained deep learning model can very accurately identify full-field digital pathological biopsy images of melanocyte-derived benign and malignant tumors. The performance of the deep learning algorithm was better than the average of 7 pathologists compared with pathologists. The deep learning algorithm can be used as an auxiliary diagnostic tool to help doctors differentiate WSI images of melanoma and nevus.

6. SUMMARY AND PROSPECT

The development of AI medicine is in full swing, which can be seen from some literature reports on AI medicine and AI pathology. Under the background that the country requires the deep integration of AI and the real economy, and based on the active implementation of medical informatization reform, big medical data, "Internet + health care" and other reform directions, the cultivation and development of medical image-assisted diagnosis system and AI medical equipment have become the development direction of AI medicine. With the help of AI medical, the medical industry will make great efforts to improve nationwide hierarchical diagnosis and treatment, scientific management and sharing of medical big data information, and construction of efficient and informationized medical services [62]. Fig. **3** showed the flow chart of AI and medical specialists in medicine.

In addition to the fierce collision of academic ideas and creativity, the field of AI medicine also faces many problems that cannot be ignored, such as the ethical problems of AI medicine, the accuracy of AI algorithm to be improved, the lack of training data caused by inconsistent medical data standards and the difficulties in collection and utilization, *etc* [63]. Digital pathology (DP), which has emerged in recent years, refers to the use of computers and networks in the field of pathology, and its core technology is full-glass digital scanning and pathology image analysis algorithm. All slides digital scanning technology (whole slide imaging, WSI) is a kind of modern digital system and the traditional optical amplification device of the organic combination of technology, it is obtained by full automatic microscope scanning acquisition of the high-resolution digital image, and application of the computer to get the image automatically and the joining together of high precision, more vision processing, quantitative pathology image information such as the shape, size, and color, to get a digital biopsy or virtual [64]. Digital slice can be used for image retrieval, pattern recognition, computer learning, and deep learning, thus laying a foundation for building a mathematical model of computer-aided diagnosis (CAD).

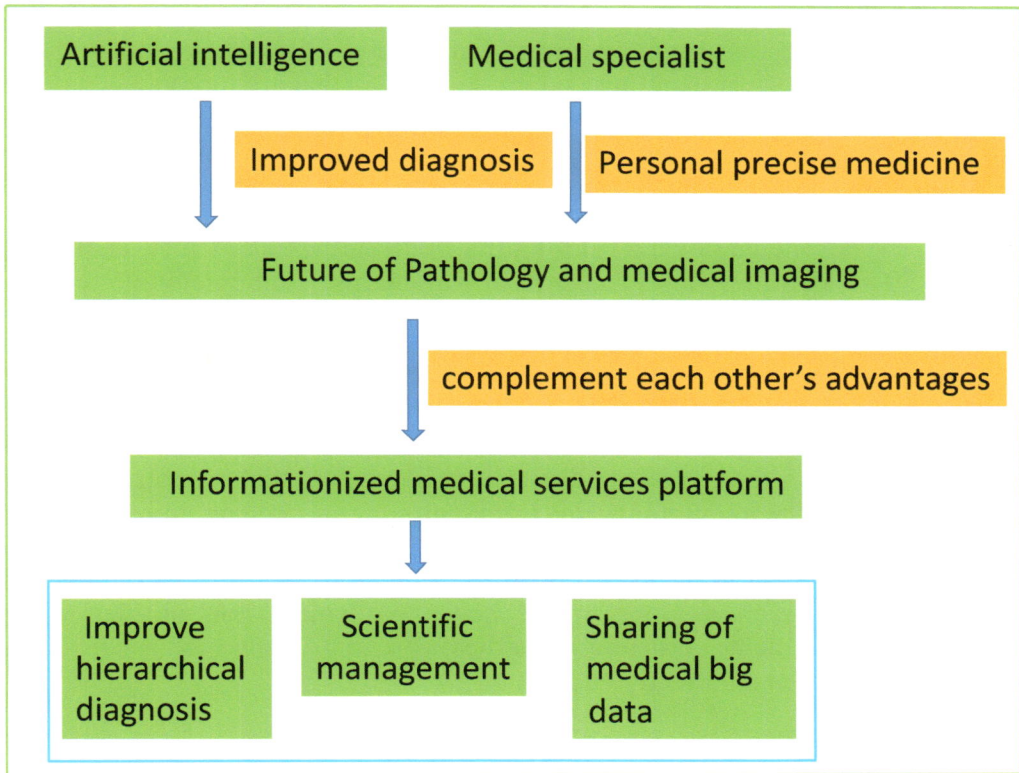

Fig. (3). The flow chart of AI and medical specialist complement the medical industry to make great efforts to improve nationwide hierarchical diagnosis and treatment, scientific management and sharing of medical big data information, and construction of efficient and informationized medical services.

WSI has broken through the limitations of traditional microscopy for pathologists. It can not only carry out remote pathological consultation *via* network transmission but also, crucially, develop CAD in combination with the constantly developing computer AI, big data, and cloud technology [65].

Several studies have shown that compared with traditional microscopy, the consistency rate of pathological diagnosis using WSI is 90% [66]. However, WSI contains a large amount of complex and redundant information, so it is necessary to filter and mine feature data before a further pathological diagnosis can be made based on the result of feature extraction. Pathology image analysis algorithm for transport, currently used are mainly the algorithm of support vector machine (support vector machine, SVM) [67] and AdaBoost and depth of convolution neural network (Convolutional neural network) [68], the task is used to solve the following three aspects: (1) feature extraction: namely, from the image selected and simplify the most can effectively express the process of low dimension vector of image content. Studies have confirmed that features of automatic learning have a better expression effect than those of manual design and are more advantageous in big data processing [69]. (2) Detection and segmentation: Traditional machine learning algorithms have limited feature presentation ability, resulting in unsatisfactory segmentation effect;

However, the advantage of deep learning lies in the automatic extraction of image features [70 - 74], which has stronger removal energy for the heterogeneity and noise of pathological sections [75].

Classification and classification: The task of pathological classification and classification is one of the important tasks in the analysis of pathological sections. The image analysis algorithm can realize classification in the high-dimensional feature space by mapping. AI medicine is a bundle of both opportunities and challenges; with the continuous development of AI medical and continuous increase in the ability to merge with medical needs, AI individual is expected to be a qualified assistant to the doctor, bear the tedious work, swallow the regional medical level differences, to promote better implementation of hierarchical diagnosis and treatment, clinical and medical research in the medical level and serve the humanity in an effective way

CONSENT FOR PUBLICATION

Not Applicable.

CONFLICT OF INTEREST

The author confirms that this chapter contents have no conflict of interest.

ACKNOWLEDGEMENT

Declared none.

REFERENCES

[1]   Weinstein RS, Graham AR, Richter LC, *et al.* Overview of telepathology, virtual microscopy, and whole slide imaging: prospects for the future. Hum Pathol 2009; 40(8): 1057-69.
        [http://dx.doi.org/10.1016/j.humpath.2009.04.006] [PMID: 19552937]

[2]   Silver D, *et al.* Mastering the game of go with deep neural networks and tree search. Nature 2017; 542: 115-8.
        [http://dx.doi.org/10.1038/nature21056] [PMID: 28117445]

[3]   Lusted LB. Logical analysis in roentgen diagnosis. Radiology 1960; 74: 178-93.
        [http://dx.doi.org/10.1148/74.2.178] [PMID: 14419034]

[4]   Awadallah MA, Morcos MM. Application of AI tools in fault diagnosis of electrical machines and drives-an overview. IEEE Trans Energ Convers 2003; 18(2): 245-51.

[http://dx.doi.org/10.1109/TEC.2003.811739]

[5]   Oehmichen M, Theuerkauf I, Meissner C. Is traumatic axonal injury (AI) associated with an early microglial activation? Application of a double-labeling technique for simultaneous detection of microglia and AI. Acta Neuropathologica 1999; 97(5): 491-4.

[6]   Hosny A, Parmar C, Quackenbush J. Artificial intelligence in radiology. Nat Rev Cancer 2018.
[http://dx.doi.org/10.1038/s41568018]

[7]   Huang S, Yang J, Fong S, Zhao Q. Artificial intelligence in cancer diagnosis and prognosis: Opportunities and challenges. Cancer Lett 2020; 471: 61-71.
[http://dx.doi.org/10.1016/j.canlet.2019.12.007] [PMID: 31830558]

[8]   Lambin P, Rios-Velazquez E, Leijenaar R, *et al.* Radiomics: extracting more information from medical images using advanced feature analysis. Eur J Cancer 2012; 48(4): 441-6.
[http://dx.doi.org/10.1016/j.ejca.2011.11.036] [PMID: 22257792]

[9]   Huang S, Yang J, Fong S, Zhao Q. Mining prognosis index of brain metastases using artificial intelligence. Cancers (Basel) 2019; 11(8): E1140.
[http://dx.doi.org/10.3390/cancers11081140] [PMID: 31395825]

[10]   Liu Bao-zhi, Li Dong-bo. Clinical Study on the Value of Artificial Intelligence (AI) in the Imaging Diagnosis of Breast Diseases. J Inner Mongolia University for Nationalities 2019; 34(5): 435-8.

[11]   Filippetti F, *et al.* AI techniques in induction machines diagnosis including the speed ripple effect. IEEE Trans Ind Appl 1998; 34(1): 98-108.
[http://dx.doi.org/10.1109/28.658729]

[12]   Bhalla D, Bansal RK, Gupta HO. Integrating AI based dga fault diagnosis using dempster–shafer theory. Int J Electr Power Energy Syst 2013; 48: 31-8.
[http://dx.doi.org/10.1016/j.ijepes.2012.11.018]

[13]   Lee H, Hong H, Kim J, Jung DC. Deep feature classification of angiomyolipoma without visible fat and renal cell carcinoma in abdominal contrast-enhanced CT images with texture image patches and hand-crafted feature concatenation. Med Phys 2018; 45(4): 1550-61.
[http://dx.doi.org/10.1002/mp.12828] [PMID: 29474742]

[14]   Narazaki H, *et al.* An AI tool and its applications to diagnosis problems. ISIJ Int 1990; 30(2): 98-104.
[http://dx.doi.org/10.2355/isijinternational.30.98]

[15]   Tim L. Clinical evaluation of atlas and deep learning based automatic contouring for lung cancer. Radiotherapy and Oncology. 2018; 126: pp. ((2))312-7.

[16]   Jia Yi Lim, Michelle L. Use of auto-segmentation in the delineation of target volumes and organs at risk in head and neck. Acta Oncologica 2016; 55(7): 799-806.

[17]   Orringer DA, *et al.* Rapid intraoperative histology of unprocessed surgical specimens *via* fibre-lase--based stimulated Raman scattering microscopy. Nat Biomed Eng 2017; 1: 0027.

[18]   Zhang J, Wang Y, Yu B, Shi X, Zhang Y. Application of computer-aided diagnosis to the sonographic evaluation of cervical lymph nodes. Ultrason Imaging 2016; 38(2): 159-71.
[http://dx.doi.org/10.1177/0161734615589080] [PMID: 26025577]

[19]   Khomfoi S, Tolbert LM. Fault diagnosis and reconfiguration for multilevel inverter drive using AI-based techniques. IEEE Trans Ind Electron 2007; 54(6): 2954-68.
[http://dx.doi.org/10.1109/TIE.2007.906994]

[20]   Haleem A, Javaid M, Khan IH. Current status and applications of artificial intelligence (AI) in medical field: an overview. Current Medicine Research and Practice 2019; 9(6): 231-7.
[http://dx.doi.org/10.1016/j.cmrp.2019.11.005]

[21]   Dordea AC, Bray MA, Allen K, *et al.* An open-source computational tool to automatically quantify immunolabeled retinal ganglion cells. Exp Eye Res 2016; 147: 50-6.
[http://dx.doi.org/10.1016/j.exer.2016.04.012] [PMID: 27119563]

[22]   Diem K, Magaret A, Klock A, Jin L, Zhu J, Corey L. Image analysis for accurately counting CD4+ and CD8+ T cells in human tissue. J Virol Methods 2015; 222: 117-21.
[http://dx.doi.org/10.1016/j.jviromet.2015.06.004] [PMID: 26073660]

[23]   Macedo ND, Buzin AR, de Araujo IB, *et al.* Automated and Reproducible Detection of Vascular Endothelial Growth Factor (VEGF) in Renal Tissue Sections. J Immunol Res 2019; 2019: 7232781.
[http://dx.doi.org/10.1155/2019/7232781] [PMID: 31016206]

[24]   Yeh FC, Parwani AV, Pantanowitz L, Ho C. Automated grading of renal cell carcinoma using whole slide imaging. J Pathol Inform 2014; 5(1): 23.
[http://dx.doi.org/10.4103/2153-3539.137726] [PMID: 25191622]

[25]   Jenneck C, Juergens U, Buecheler M, Novak N. Pathogenesis, diagnosis, and treatment of aspirin intolerance. Ann Allergy Asthma Immunol 2007; 99(1): 13-21.
[http //dx.doi.org/10.1016/S1081-1206(10)60615-1] [PMID: 17650824]

[26]   Xiong Y, Ba X, Hou A, Zhang K, Chen L, Li T. Automatic detection of mycobacterium tuberculosis using artificial intelligence. J Thorac Dis 2018; 10(3): 1936-40.
[http://dx.doi.org/10.21037/jtd.2018.01.91] [PMID: 29707349]

[27]   Sheikhzadeh F, Ward RK, van Niekerk D, Guillaud M. Automatic labeling of molecular biomarkers of immunohistochemistry images using fully convolutional networks. PLoS One 2018; 13(1): e0190783.
[http://dx.doi.org/10.1371/journal.pone.0190783] [PMID: 29351281]

[28]   Yu K-H, Zhang C, Berry GJ, *et al.* Predicting non-small cell lung cancer prognosis by fully automated microscopic pathology image features. Nat Commun 2016; 7(1): 12474.
[http://dx.doi.org/10.1038/ncomms12474] [PMID: 27527408]

[29]   Huang S, Yang J, Fong S, Zhao Q. Mining prognosis index of brain metastases using artificial intelligence. Cancers (Basel) 2019; 11(8): E1140.
[http://dx.doi.org/10.3390/cancers11081140] [PMID: 31395825]

[30]   Burki TK. Predicting lung cancer prognosis using machine learning. Lancet Oncol 2016; 17(10): e421.
[http://dx.doi.org/10.1016/S1470-2045(16)30436-3] [PMID: 27569440]

[31]   Beck AH, Sangoi AR, Leung S, *et al.* Systematic analysis of breast cancer morphology uncovers stromal features associated with survival Sci Transl Med 2011; 3(108): 108ra113.
[http://dx.doi.org/10.1126/scitranslmed.3002564]

[33]   Huang S, Yang J, Fong S, Zhao Q. Mining prognosis index of brain metastases using artificial intelligence. Cancers (Basel) 2019; 11(8): E1140.
[http://dx.doi.org/10.3390/cancers11081140] [PMID: 31395825]

[34]   Beck AH, Sangoi AR, Leung S, *et al.* Systematic analysis of breast cancer morphology uncovers stromal features associated with survival. Sci Transl Med 2011; 3(108): 108ra113.

[35]   Ichimasa K, Shin-Ei Kudo, Mori Y, *et al.* Artificial intelligence may help in predicting the need for additional surgery after endoscopic resection of T1 colorectal cancer. Endoscopy 2018; 50(3): 294-5.
[PMID: 29482251]

[36]   Kwak M. Single cell functional analysis: from hematopoietic cancer to autoimmunity. Yale University 2017.

[37]   Yu KH, Zhang C, Berry GJ, *et al.* Predicting non-small cell lung cancer prognosis by fully automated microscopic pathology image features. Nat Commun 2016; 7: 12474.
[http://dx.doi.org/10.1038/ncomms12474] [PMID: 27527408]

[38]   Burridge PW, Li YF, Matsa E, *et al.* Human induced pluripotent stem cell-derived cardiomyocytes recapitulate the predilection of breast cancer patients to doxorubicin-induced cardiotoxicity. Nat Med 2016; 22(5): 547-56.
[http://dx.doi.org/10.1038/nm.4087] [PMID: 27089514]

[39]   Kumar U, *et al.* Deep learning for healthcare biometrics. Design and Implementation of Healthcare

Biometric Systems. IGI Global 2019; pp. 73-108.
[http://dx.doi.org/10.4018/978-1-5225-7525-2.ch004]

[40]   Brinker TJ, Hekler A, Enk AH, *et al.* Collaborators. Deep learning outperformed 136 of 157 dermatologists in a head-to-head dermoscopic melanoma image classification task. Eur J Cancer 2019; 113: 47-54.
[http://dx.doi.org/10.1016/j.ejca.2019.04.001] [PMID: 30981091]

[41]   Madabhushi A, *et al.* Automatic detection of mitosis using handcrafted and convolutional neural network features. Google Patents 2016.

[42]   Lu C. Computer-aided Analysis of Whole Slide Skin Histopathological Images. Canada: University of Alberta 2013.

[43]   Henschel L, Conjeti S, Estrada S, Diers K, Fischl B, Reuter M. FastSurfer - A fast and accurate deep learning based neuroimaging pipeline. Neuroimage 2020; 219: 117012.
[http://dx.doi.org/10.1016/j.neuroimage.2020.117012] [PMID: 32526386]

[44]   Trifas AM. Medical image enhancement 2005.

[45]   Wei B. Differential diagnosis of melanoma tumor pathologic images based on deep learning algorithm 2019.

[46]   Hansda G. Super-Resolution with Better Edge Enhancement 2013.

[47]   Doyle S. Computerized detection, segmentation and classification of digital pathology: Case study in prostate cancer. Rutgers The State University of New Jersey-New Brunswick and University of 2011.

[48]   Zhao X, Wang P, Tao X, Zhong N. Genetic services and testing in China. J Community Genet 2013; 4(3): 379-90.
[http://dx.doi.org/10.1007/s12687-013-0144-2] [PMID: 23595912]

[49]   Qiu W-Q, Shi JF, Guo LW, *et al.* Medical expenditure for liver cancer in urban China: A 10-year multicenter retrospective survey (2002-2011). J Cancer Res Ther 2018; 14(1): 163-70.
[http://dx.doi.org/10.4103/jcrt.JCRT_709_16] [PMID: 29516981]

[50]   Hillier SM, Jewell T. Health care and traditional medicine in China 1800-1982. Routledge 2013.
[http://dx.doi.org/10.4324/9781315018768]

[51]   Simoes P. Treatment outcomes for Hodgkin's lymphoma patients aged 60 and older: A report from the Brazilian perspective Hodgkin's lymphoma registry. Haematologica 2016.

[52]   De Fauw J, Ledsam JR, Romera-Paredes B, *et al.* Clinically applicable deep learning for diagnosis and referral in retinal disease. Nat Med 2018; 24(9): 1342-50.
[http://dx.doi.org/10.1038/s41591-018-0107-6] [PMID: 30104768]

[53]   Zhang F, *et al.* Multi-modal deep learning model for auxiliary diagnosis of Alzheimer's disease. Neurocomputing 2019; 361: 185-95.
[http://dx.doi.org/10.1016/j.neucom.2019.04.093]

[54]   Qureshi MNI, Oh J, Cho D, Jo HJ, Lee B. Multimodal discrimination of schizophrenia using hybrid weighted feature concatenation of brain functional connectivity and anatomical features with an extreme learning machine. Front Neuroinform 2017; 11: 59.
[http://dx.doi.org/10.3389/fninf.2017.00059] [PMID: 28943848]

[55]   Oh SL, Ng EYK, Tan RS, Acharya UR. Automated diagnosis of arrhythmia using combination of CNN and LSTM techniques with variable length heart beats. Comput Biol Med 2018; 102: 278-87.
[http://dx.doi.org/10.1016/j.compbiomed.2018.06.002] [PMID: 29903630]

[56]   Chen Z, *et al.* Deep residual network based fault detection and diagnosis of photovoltaic arrays using current-voltage curves and ambient conditions. Energy Convers Manage 2019; 198: 111793.
[http://dx.doi.org/10.1016/j.enconman.2019.111793]

[57]   Mardani M, Gong E, Cheng JY, *et al.* Deep generative adversarial neural networks for compressive

sensing MRI. IEEE Trans Med Imaging 2019; 38(1): 167-79.
[http://dx.doi.org/10.1109/TMI.2018.2858752] [PMID: 30040634]

[58]   Lo Y-C, *et al.* Glomerulus detection on light microscopic images of renal pathology with the faster R-CNN. International Conference on Neural Information Processing.
[http://dx.doi.org/10.1007/978-3-030-04239-4_33]

[59]   Jafari-Marandi R, *et al.* An optimum ANN-based breast cancer diagnosis: Bridging gaps between ANN learning and decision-making goals. Appl Soft Comput 2018; 72: 108-20.
[http://dx.doi.org/10.1016/j.asoc.2018.07.060]

[60]   Rezvantalab A, Safigholi H, Karimijeshni S. Dermatologist level dermoscopy skin cancer classification using different deep learning convolutional neural networks algorithms. arXiv preprint arXiv:181010348 2018.2018.

[61]   Jen K-Y, Olson JL, Brodsky S, Zhou XJ, Nadasdy T, Laszik ZG. Reliability of whole slide images as a diagnostic modality for renal allograft biopsies. Hum Pathol 2013; 44(5): 888-94.
[http://dx.doi.org/10.1016/j.humpath.2012.08.015] [PMID: 23199528]

[62]   El Achi H, Khoury JD. Artificial Intelligence and Digital Microscopy Applications in Diagnostic Hematopathology. Cancers (Basel) 2020; 12(4): 797.
[http://dx.doi.org/10.3390/cancers12040797] [PMID: 32224980]

[63]   Kowsari K, Diagnosis and analysis of celiac disease and environmental enteropathy on biopsy images using deep learning approaches. arXiv preprint arXiv:2006.06627, 2020.

[64]   Wang X, *et al.* Weakly Supervised Deep Learning for Whole Slide Lung Cancer Image Analysis. IEEE Trans Cybern 2019.
[http://dx.doi.org/10.1109/TCYB.2019.2935141] [PMID: 31484154]

[65]   Parwani AV. Digital pathology as a platform for primary diagnosis and augmentation *via* deep learning. Artificial Intelligence and Deep Learning in Pathology. Elsevier. p. 93-118.

[66]   Saltz J, *et al.* Spatial organization and molecular correlation of tumor-infiltrating lymphocytes using deep learning on pathology images 2018.
[http://dx.doi.org/10.1016/j.celrep.2018.03.086]

[67]   Serag A, Ion-Margineanu A, Qureshi H, *et al.* Translational AI and deep learning in diagnostic pathology. Front Med (Lausanne) 2019; 6: 185.
[http://dx.doi.org/10.3389/fmed.2019.00185] [PMID: 31632973]

[68]   Levine AB, Schlosser C, Grewal J, Coope R, Jones SJM, Yip S. Rise of the machines: Advances in deep learning for cancer diagnosis. Trends Cancer 2019; 5(3): 157-69.
[http://dx.doi.org/10.1016/j.trecan.2019.02.002] [PMID: 30898263]

[69]   Cho K-O, Lee SH, Jang H-J. Feasibility of fully automated classification of whole slide images based on deep learning. Korean J Physiol Pharmacol 2020; 24(1): 89-99.
[http://dx.doi.org/10.4196/kjpp.2020.24.1.89] [PMID: 31908578]

[70]   Hu Q, Yang J, Qin P, Fong S. Towards a Context-Free Machine Universal Grammar (CF-MUG) in Natural Language Processing. IEEE Access 2020; 8: 165111-29.
[http://dx.doi.org/10.1109/ACCESS.2020.3022674]

[71]   J. Yang, S.G. Huang, R. Tang, e. al., Broad Learning with Attribute Selection for Rheumatoid Arthritis, in: IEEE International Conference on Systems, Man and Cybernetics (SMC), IEEE, Toronto, 2020.

[72]   Hu Q, Yang J, Qin P, Fong S, Guo J. Could or could not of Grid-Loc: grid BLE structure for indoor localisation system using machine learning. Serv Oriented Comput Appl 2020.
[http://dx.doi.org/10.1007/s11761-020-00292-z]

[73]   Yang J, Fong S, Li T. Attribute reduction based on multi-objective decomposition-ensemble optimizer with rough set and entropy. International Conference on Data Mining Workshops (ICDMW) 2019;

673-80.

[74]   Huang S, Yang J, Fong S, Zhao Q. Artificial intelligence in cancer diagnosis and prognosis: Opportunities and challenges. Cancer Lett 2020; 471: 61-71.
[http://dx.doi.org/10.1016/j.canlet.2019.12.007] [PMID: 31830558]

[75]   Feng M, Deng Y, Yang L, *et al.* Automated quantitative analysis of Ki-67 staining and HE images recognition and registration based on whole tissue sections in breast carcinoma. Diagn Pathol 2020; 15(1): 65.
[http://dx.doi.org/10.1186/s13000-020-00957-5] [PMID: 32471471]

SUBJECT INDEX

www.ingramcontent.com/pod-product-compliance
Lightning Source LLC
Chambersburg PA
CBHW041712210326
41598CB00007B/621